THE
100 MOST BEAUTIFUL
PAINTINGS
of
BIRDS

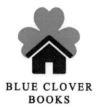

**BLUE CLOVER
BOOKS**

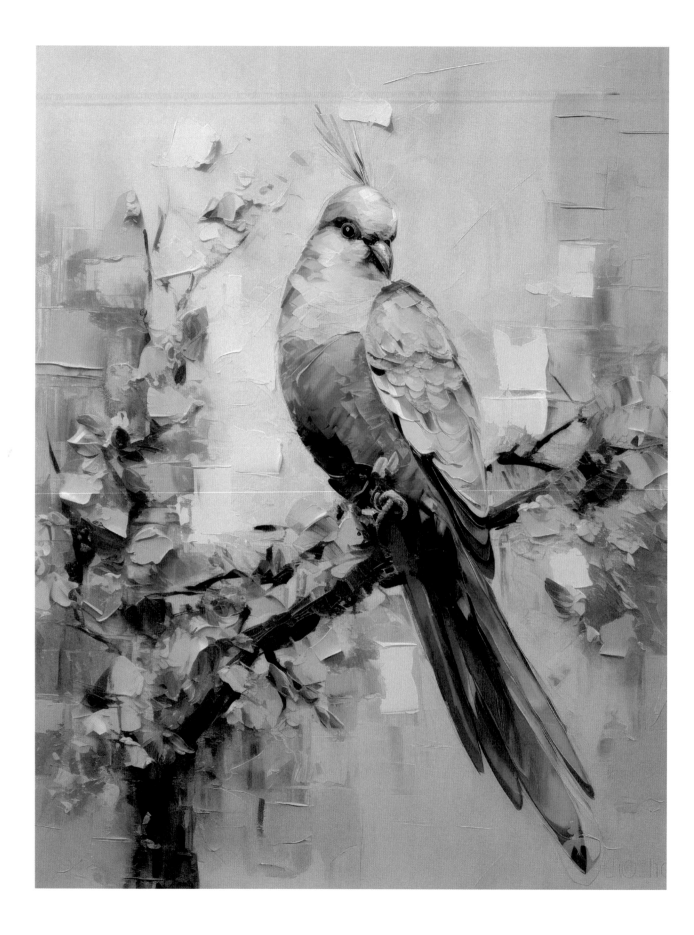

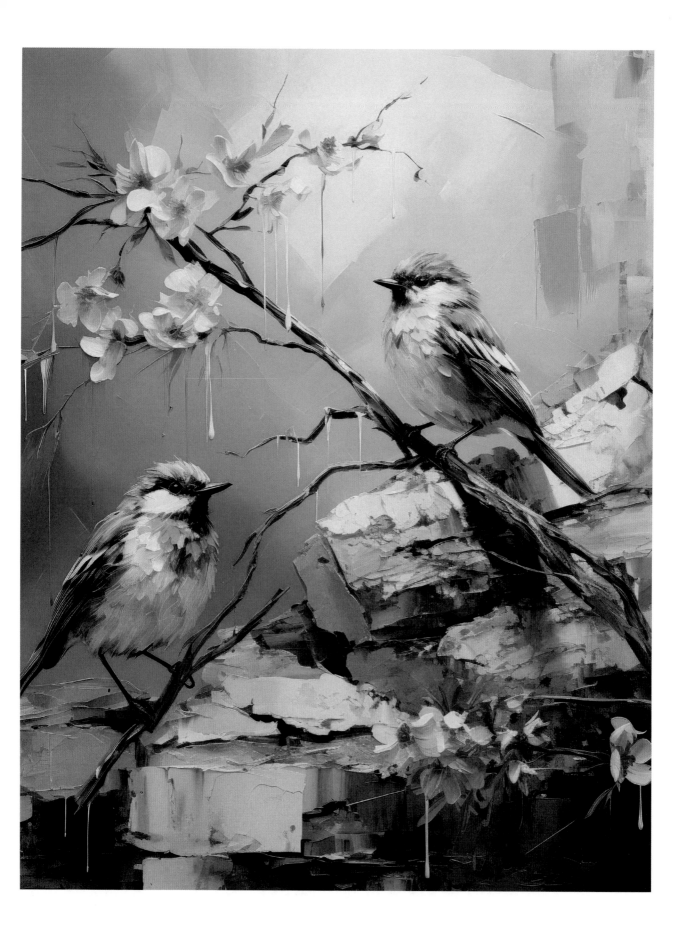

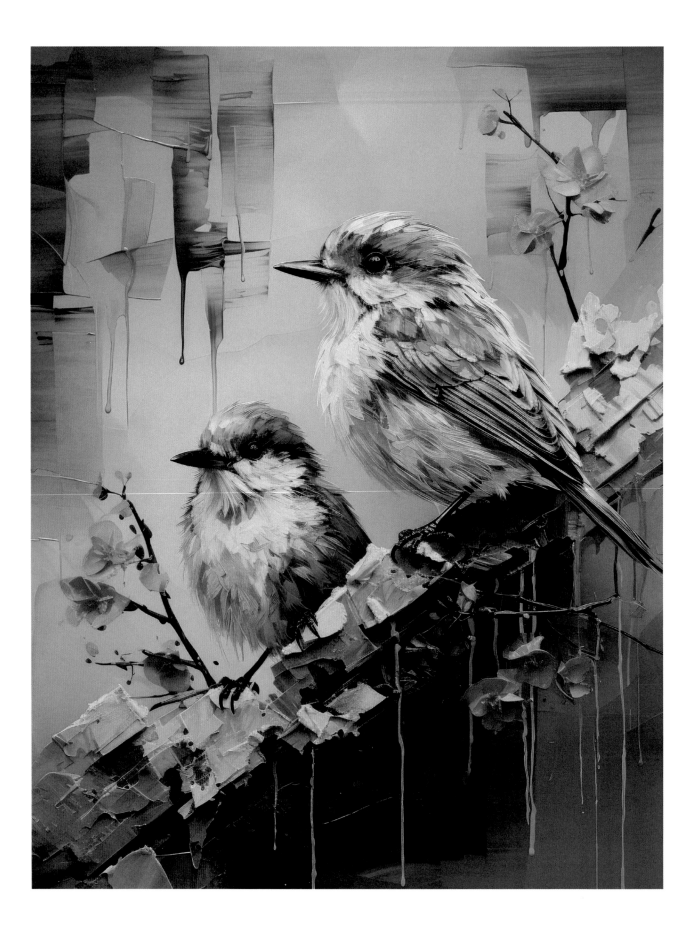

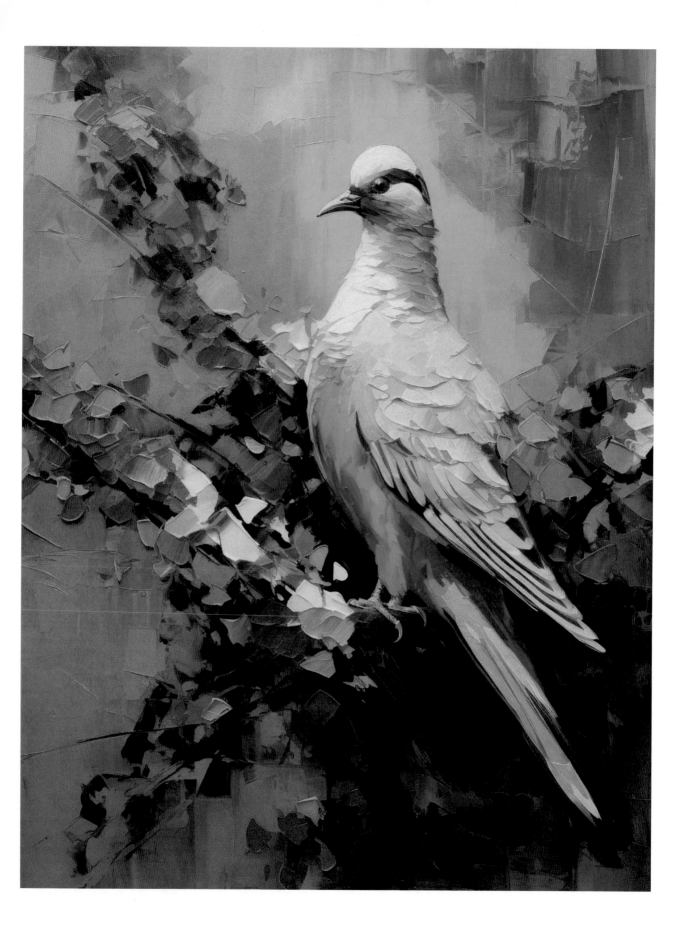

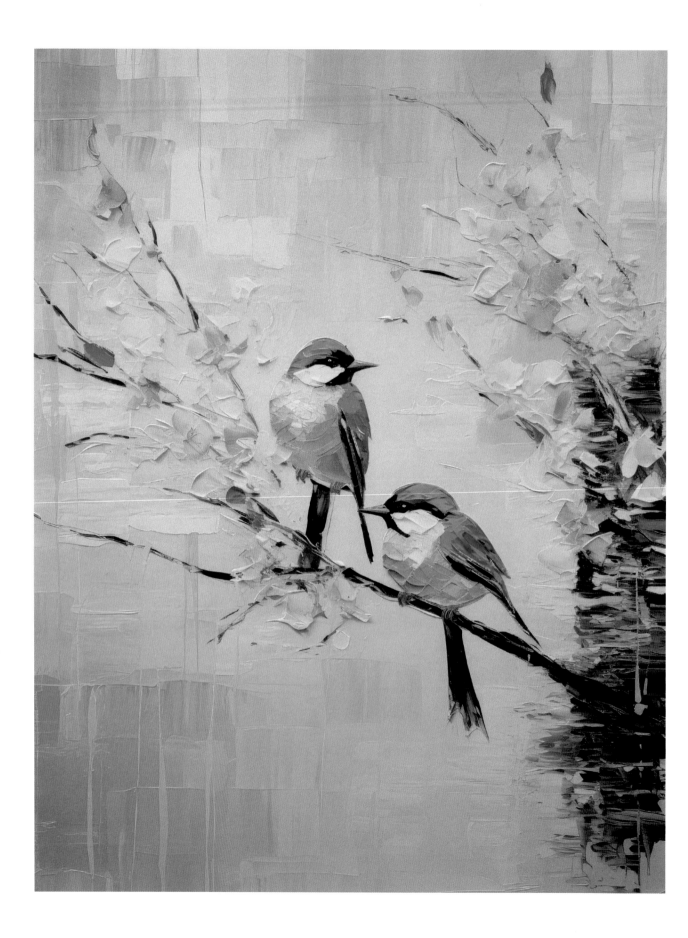

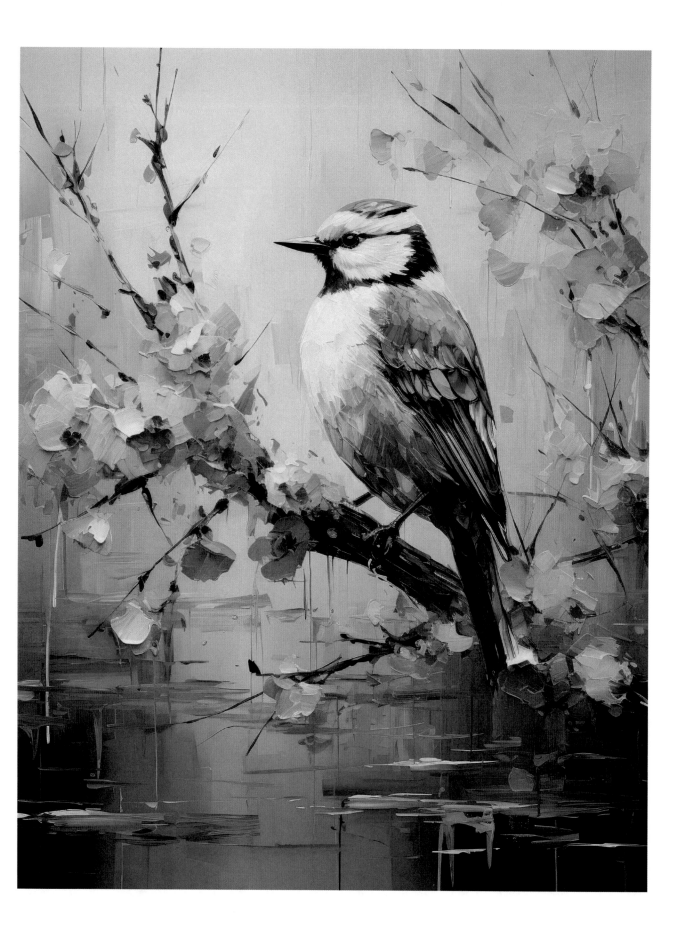

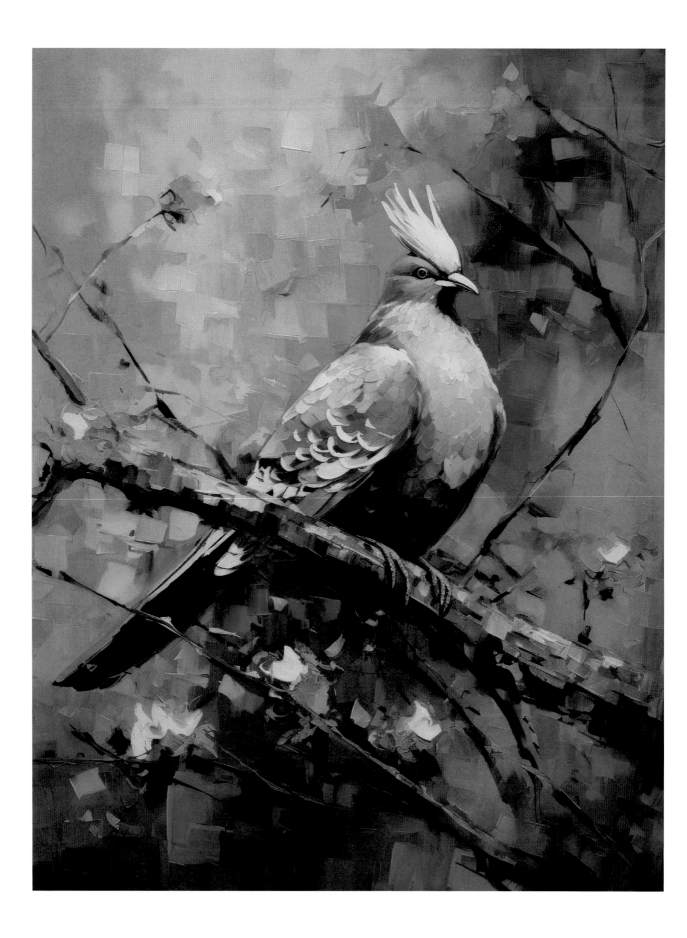

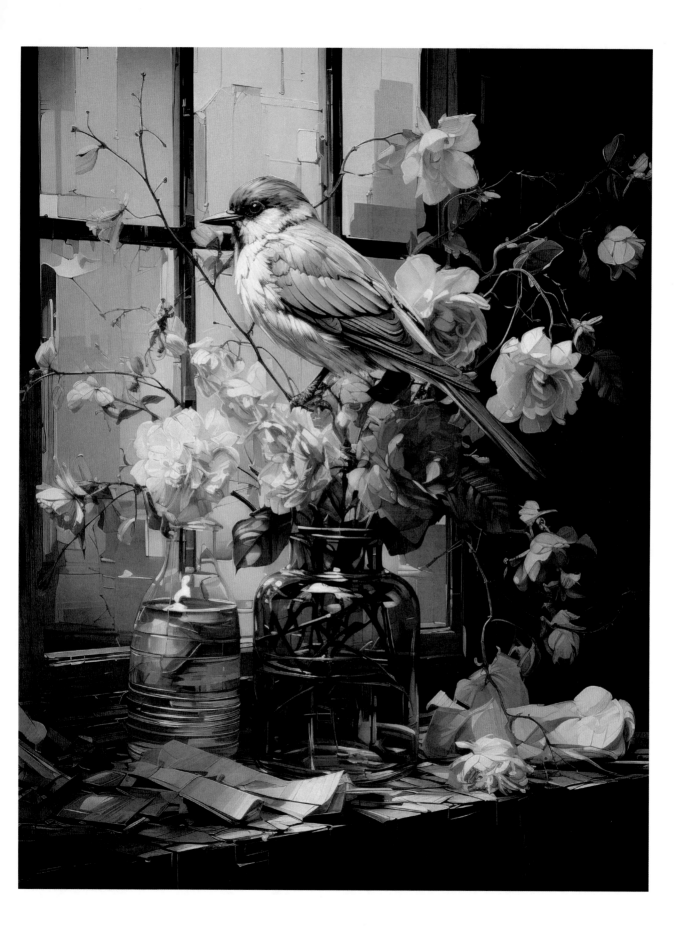

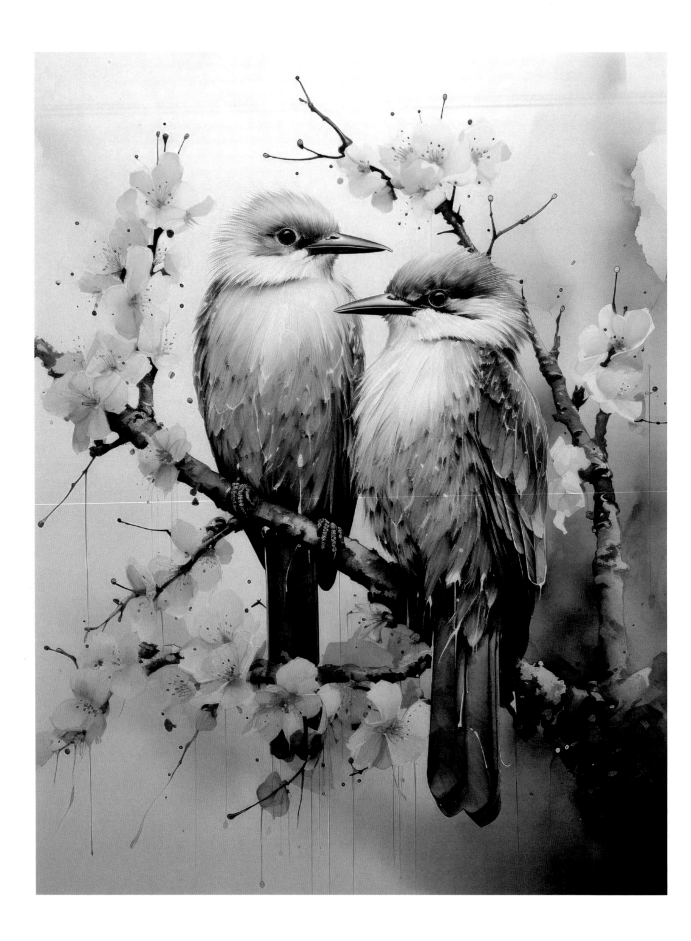

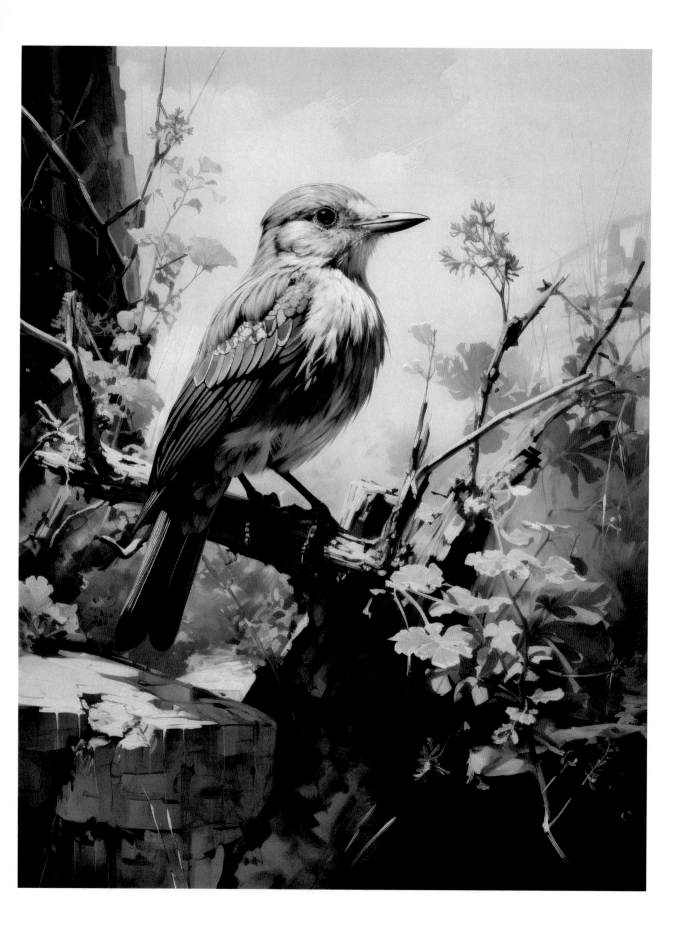

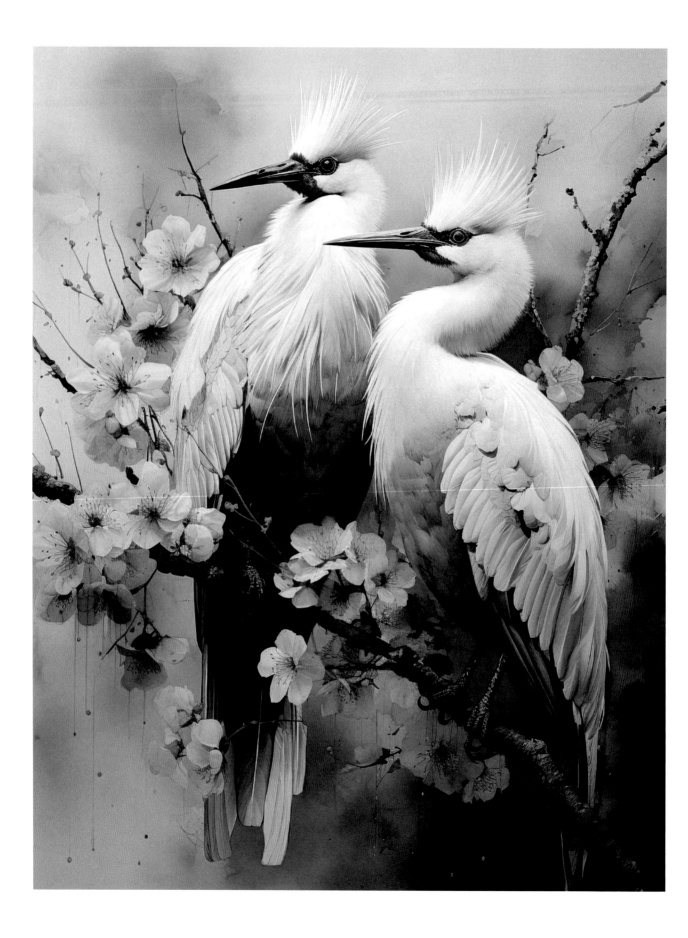

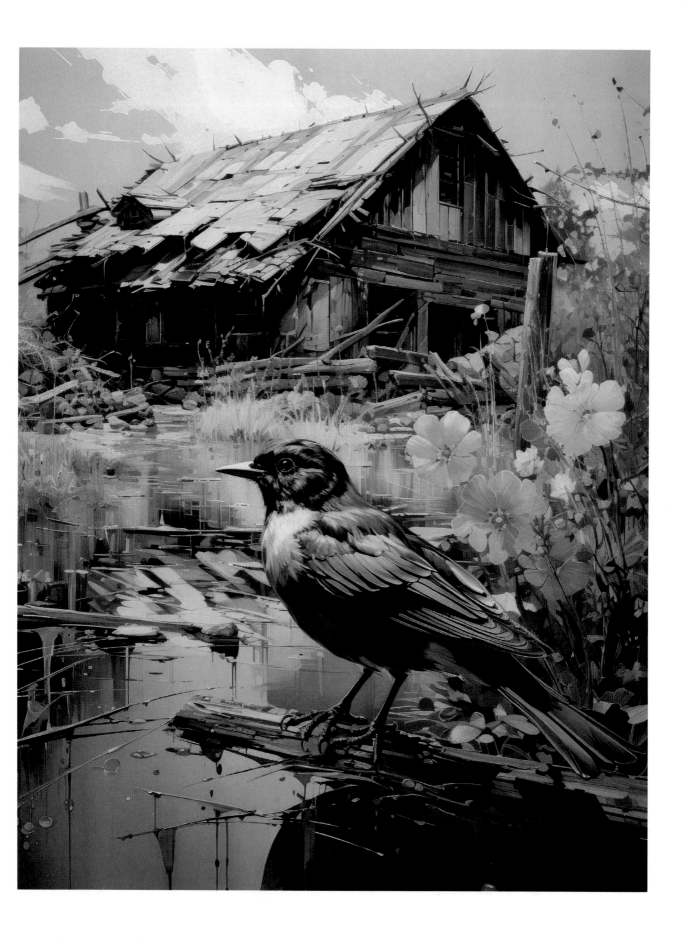

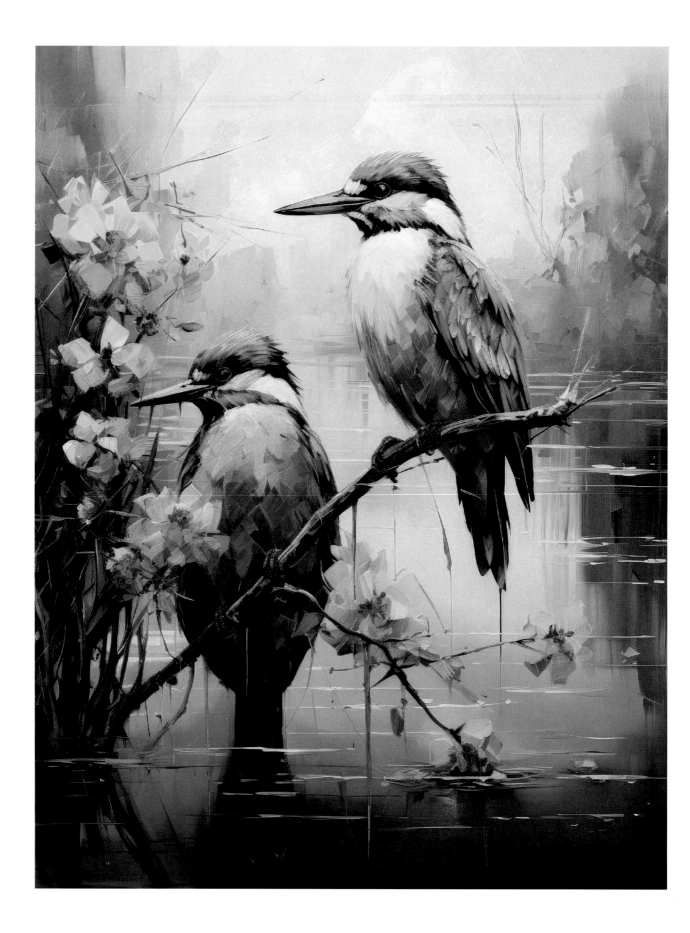

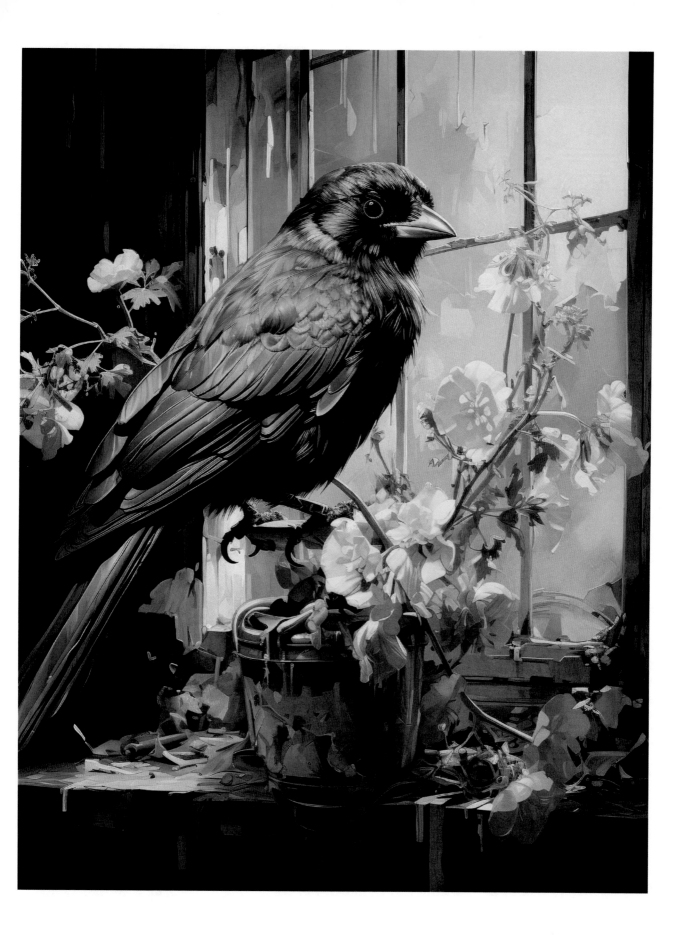

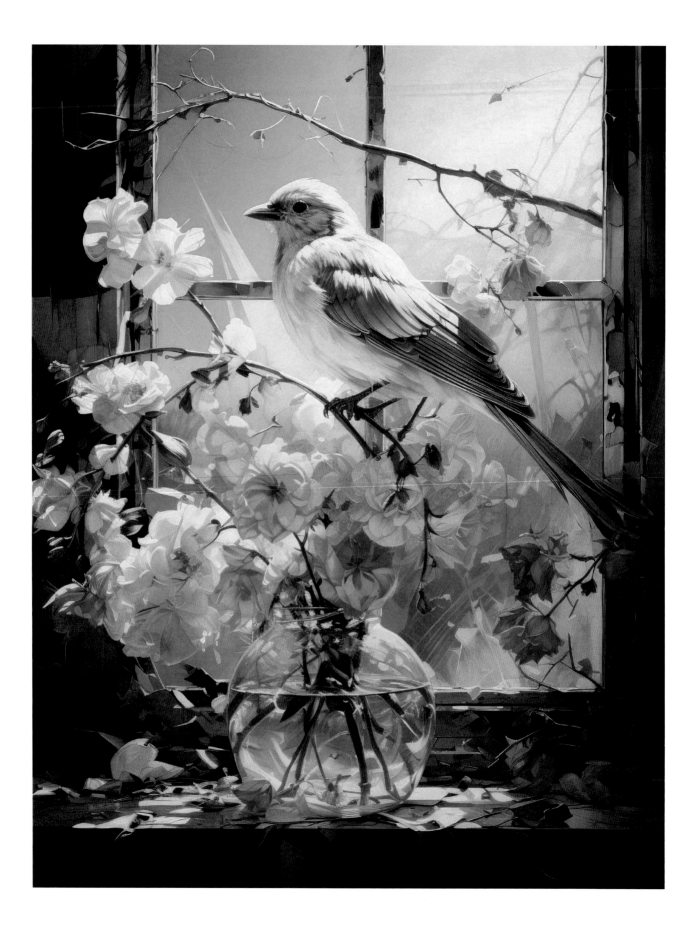

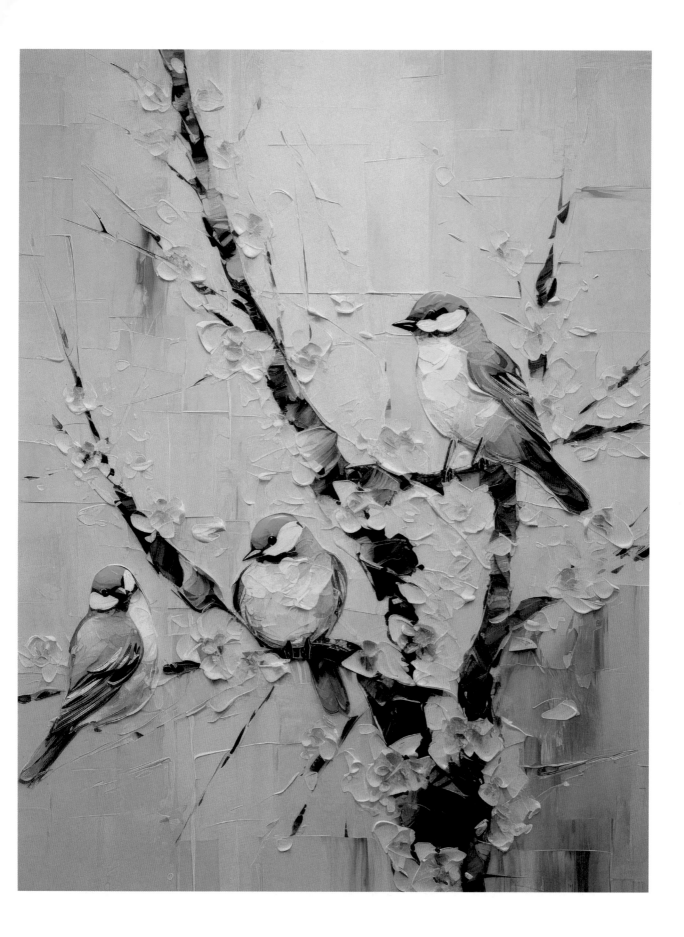

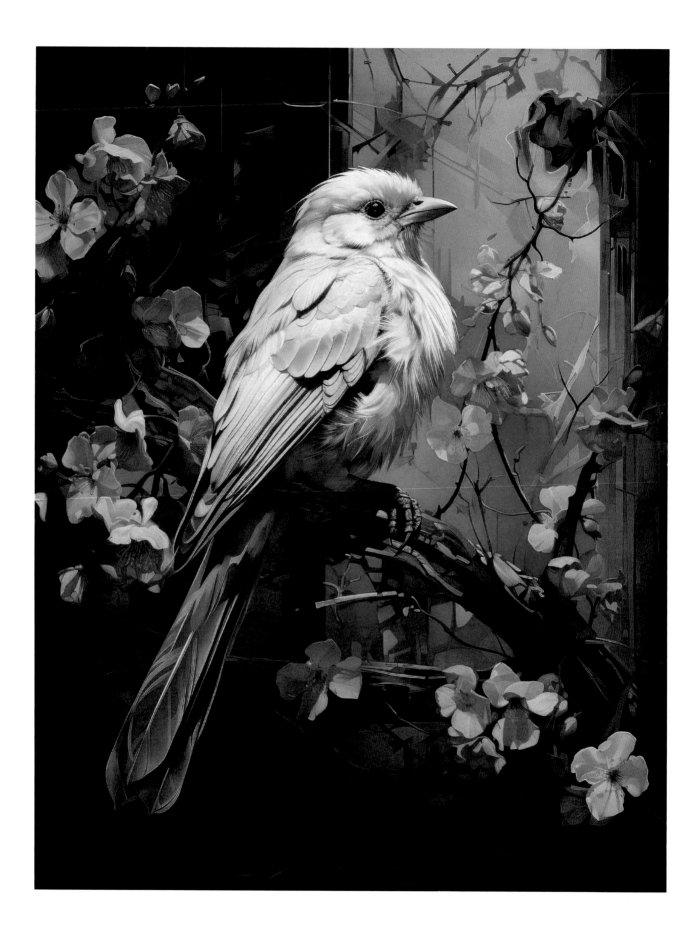

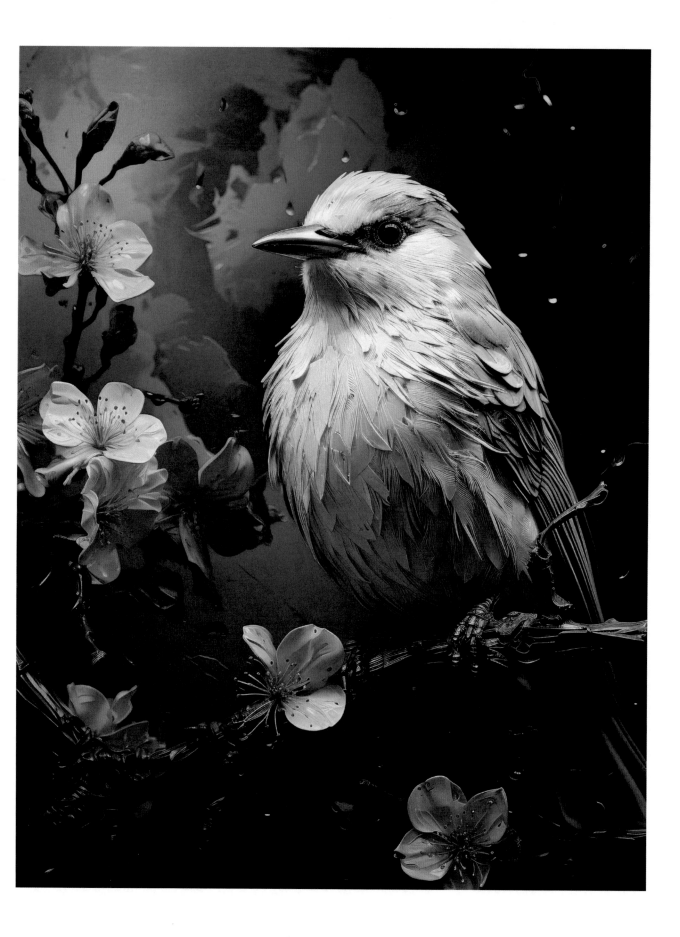

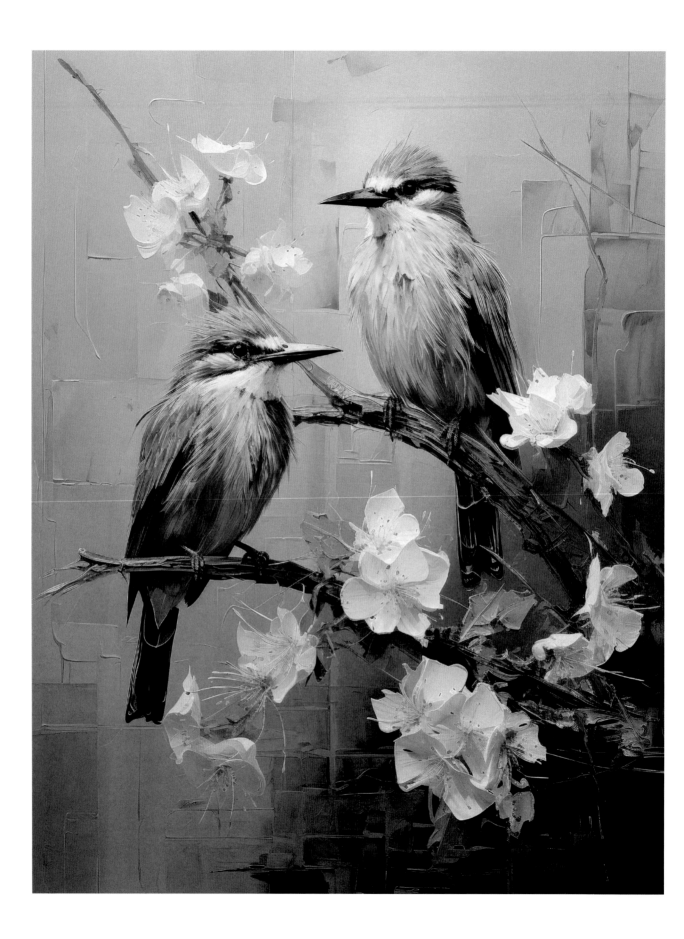

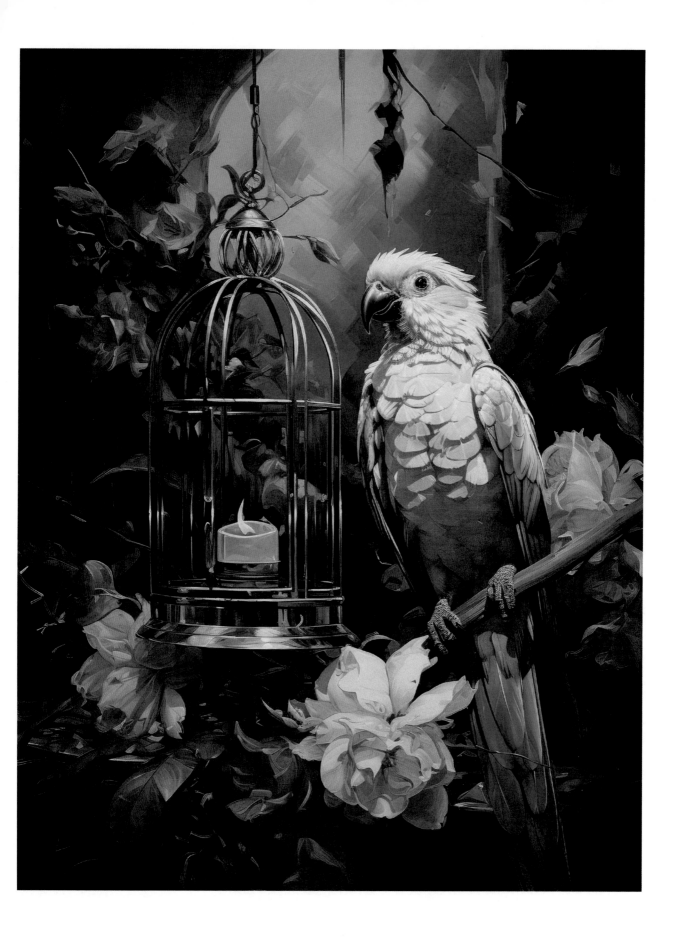

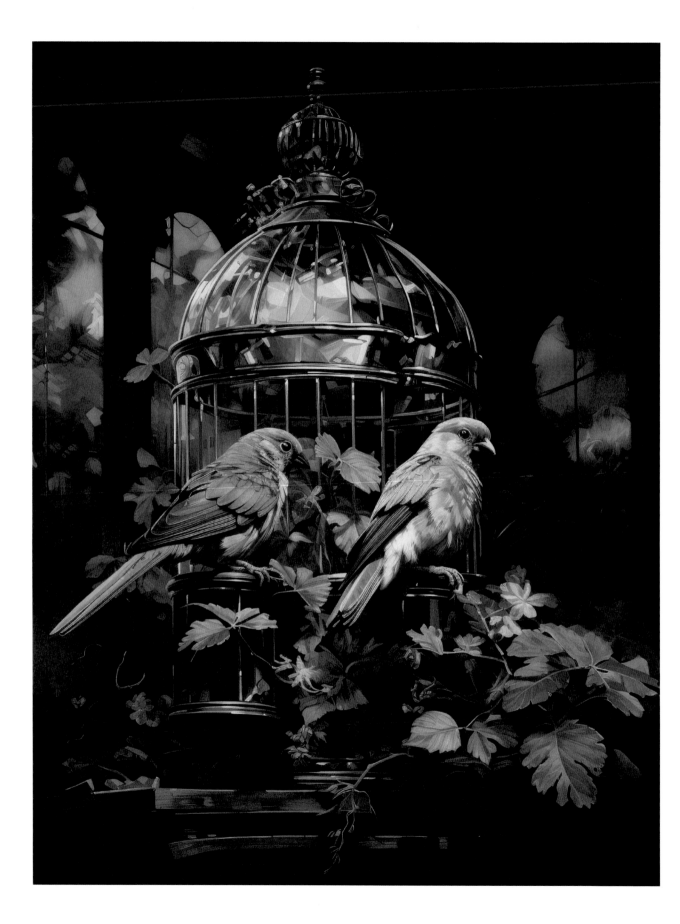

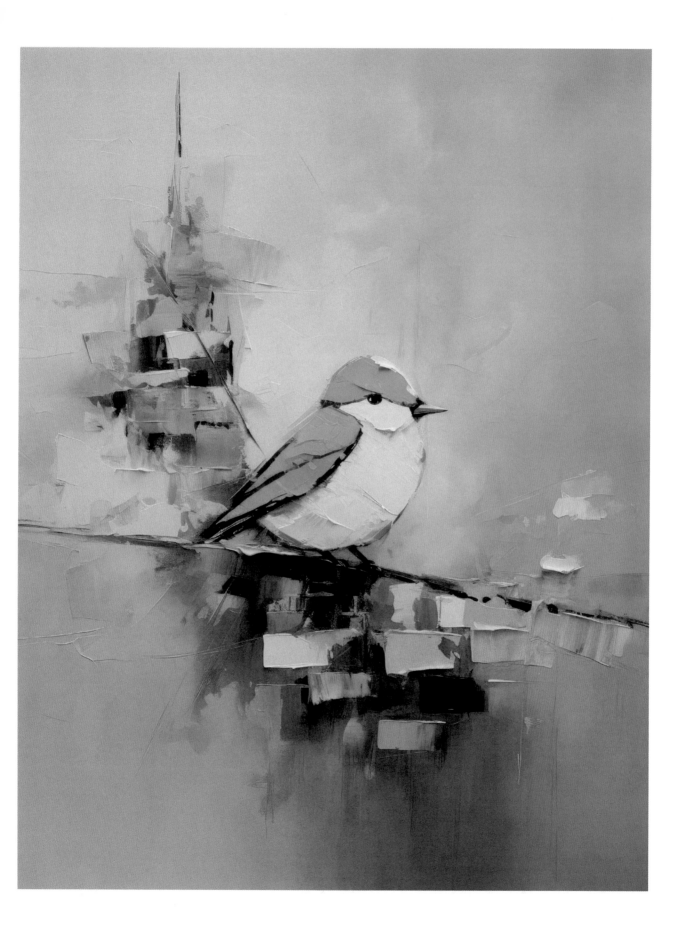

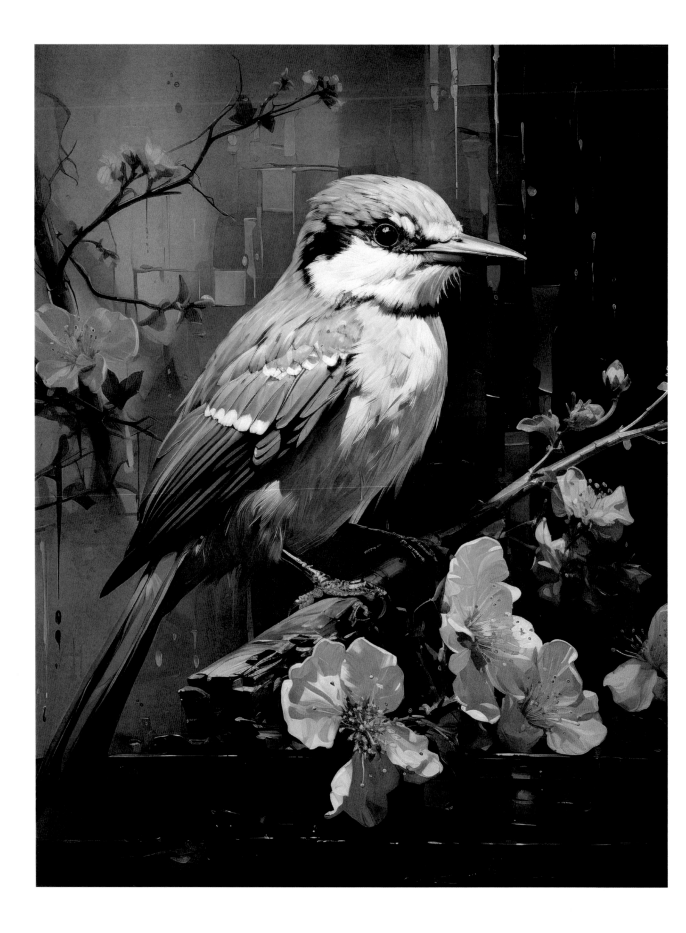

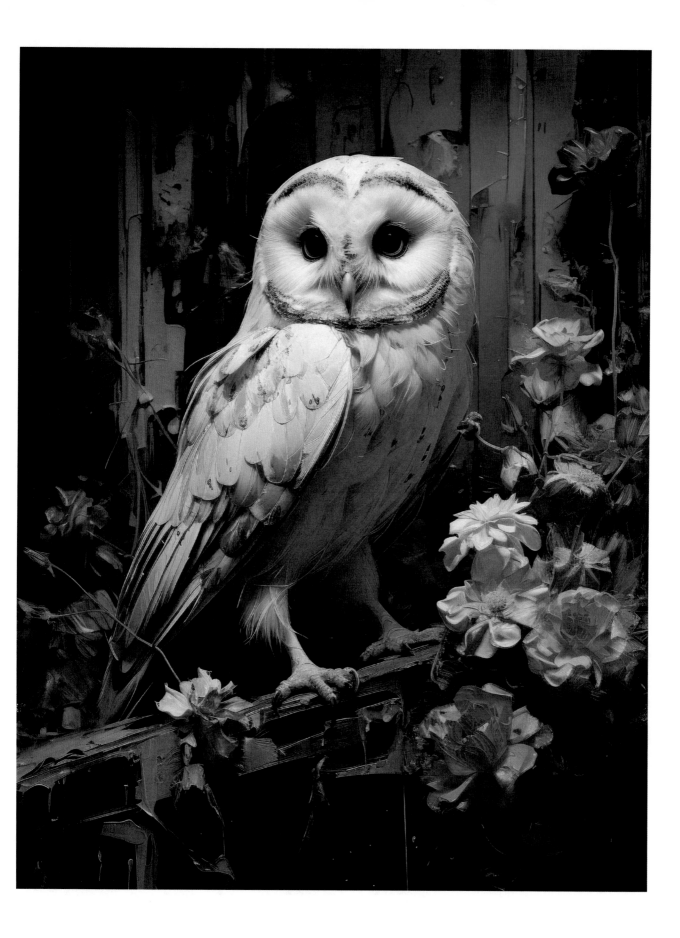

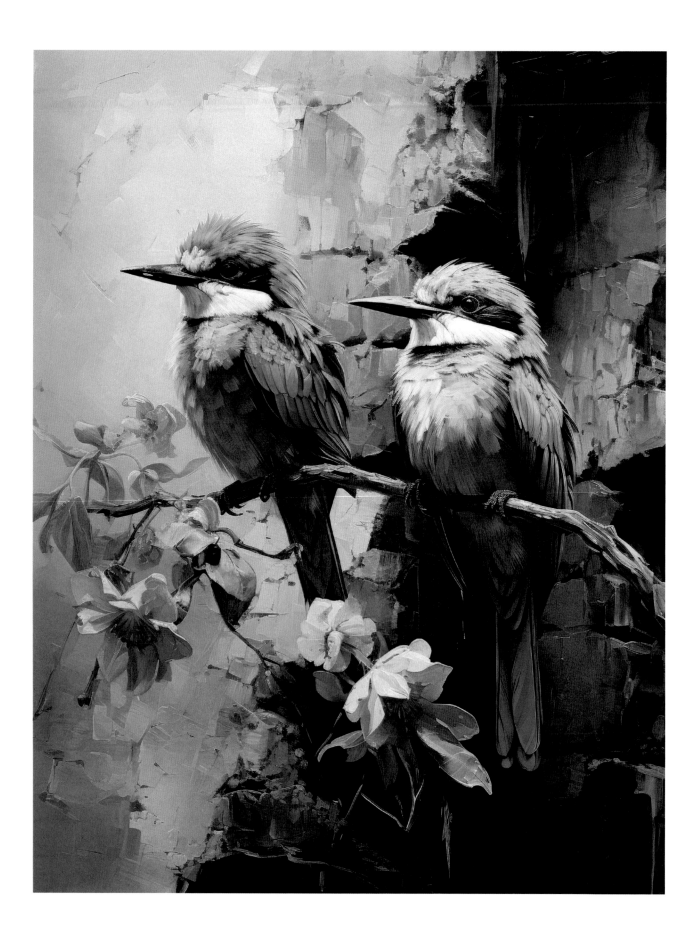

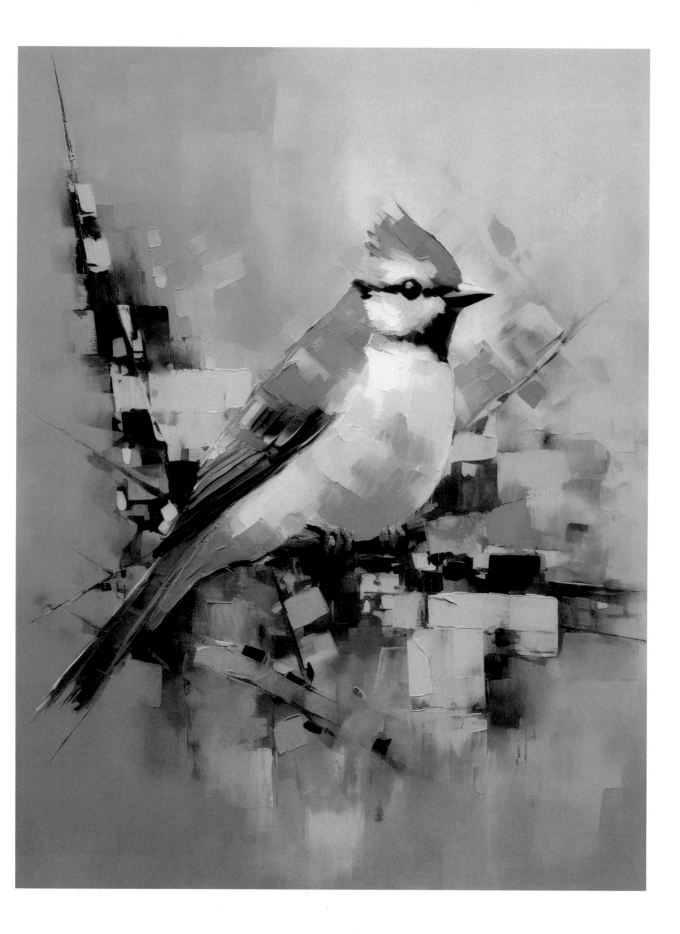

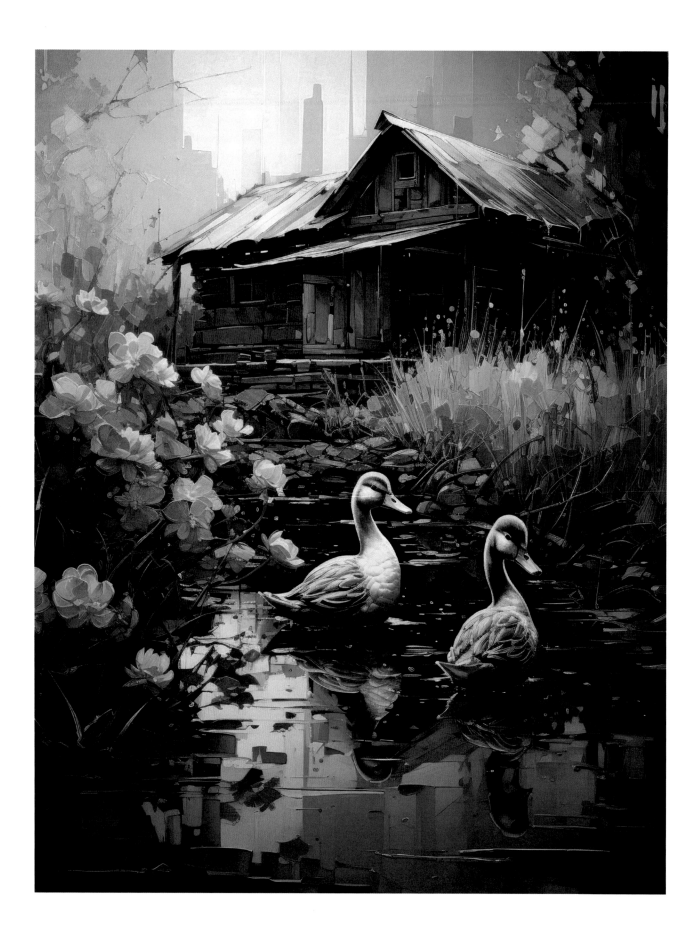

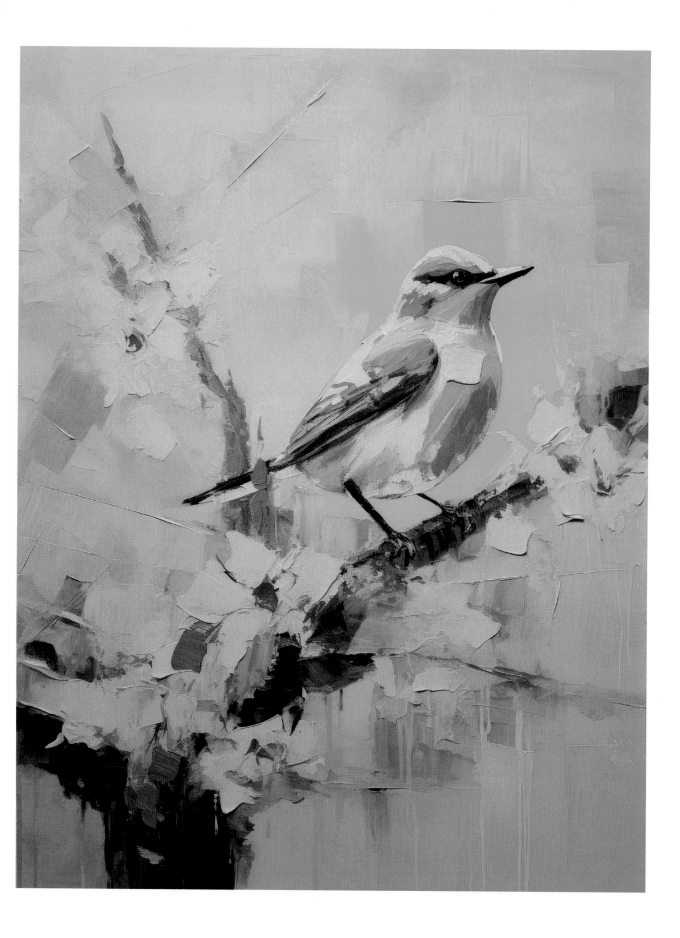

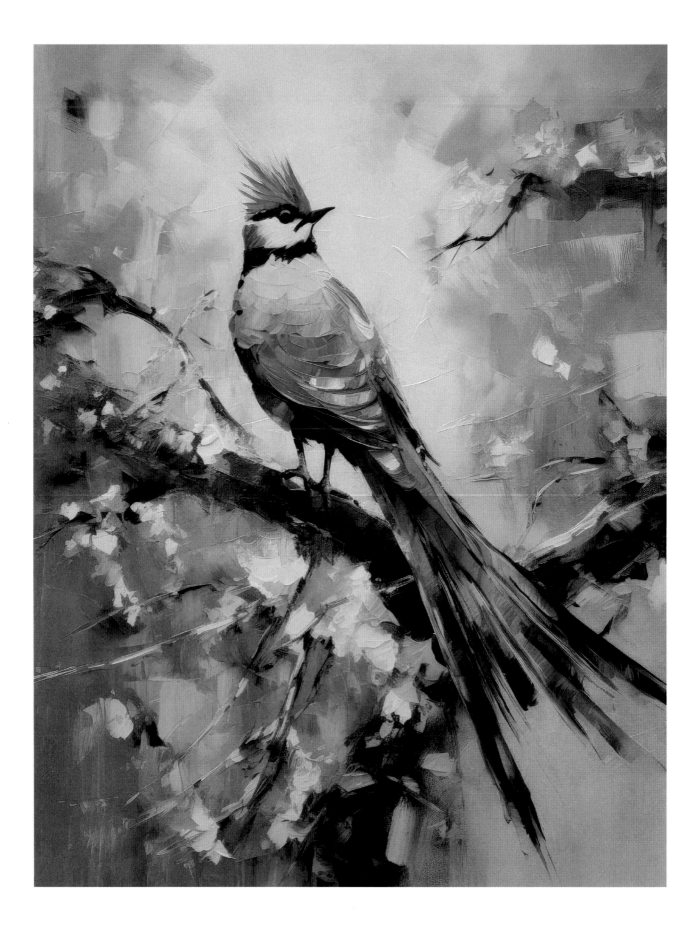

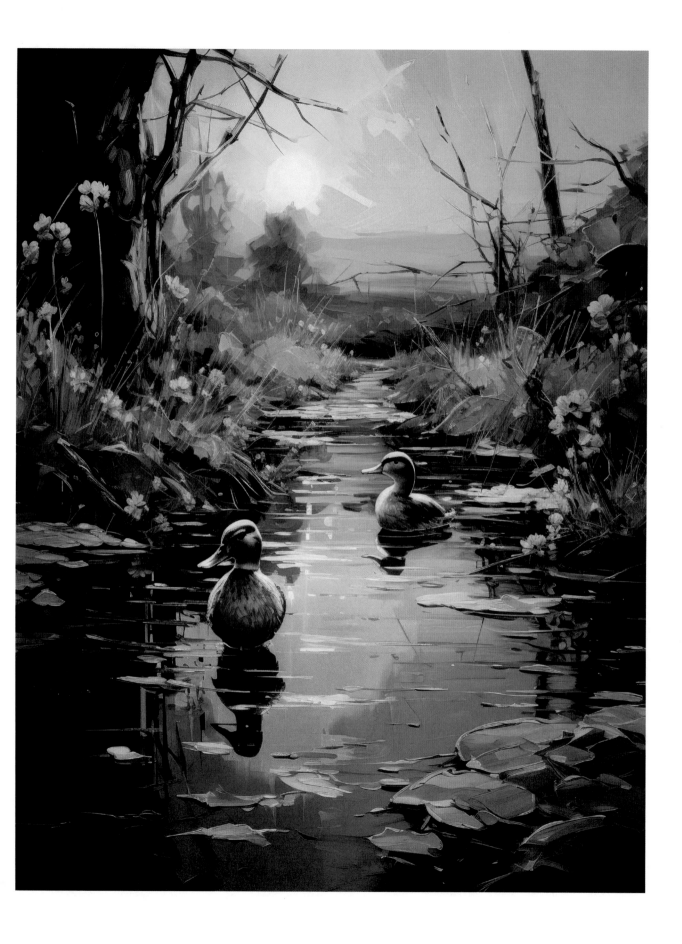

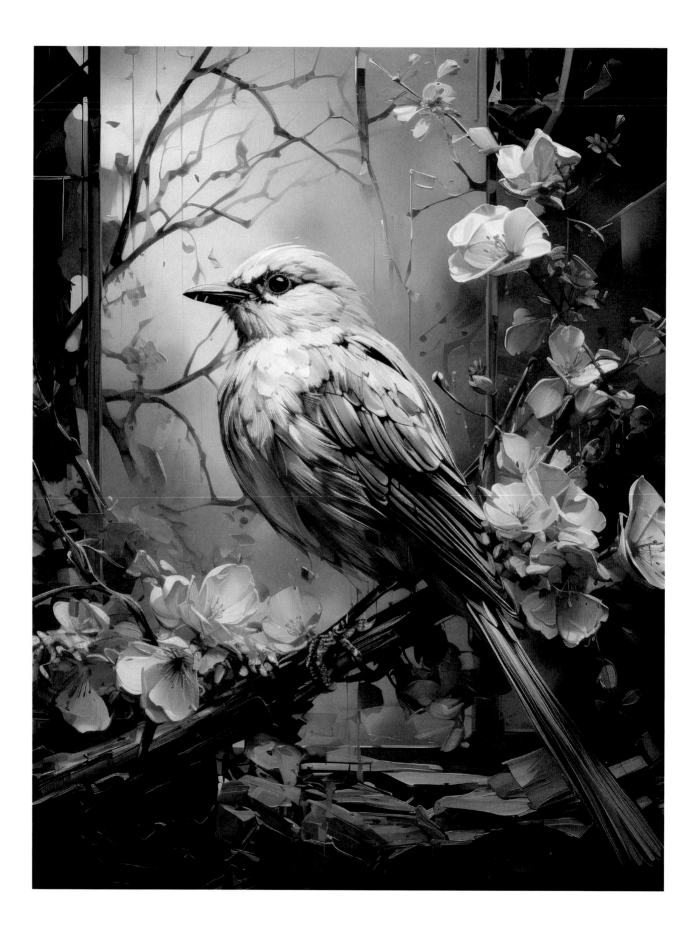

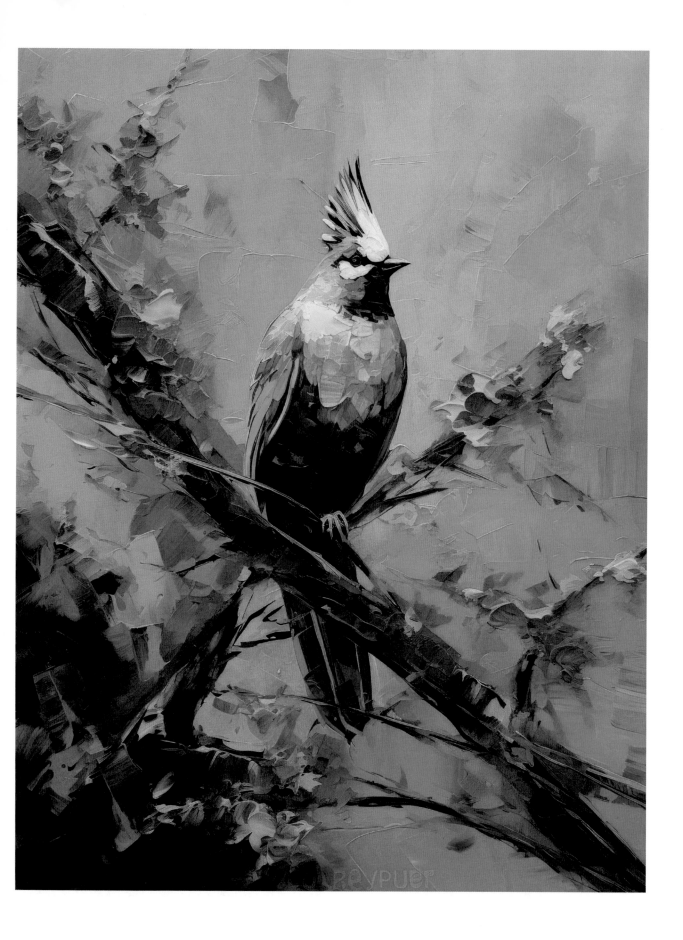

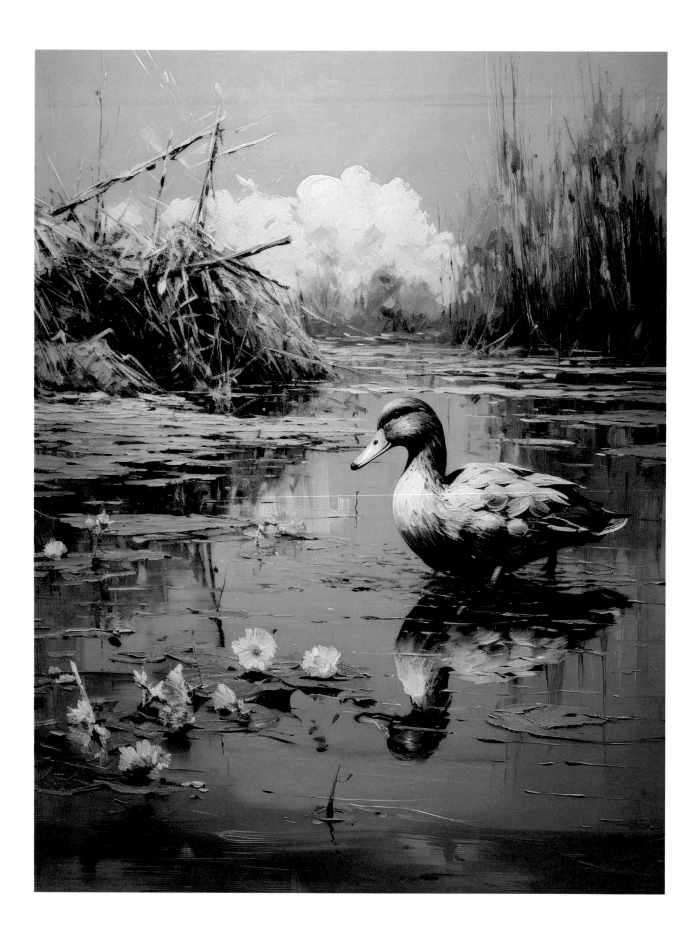

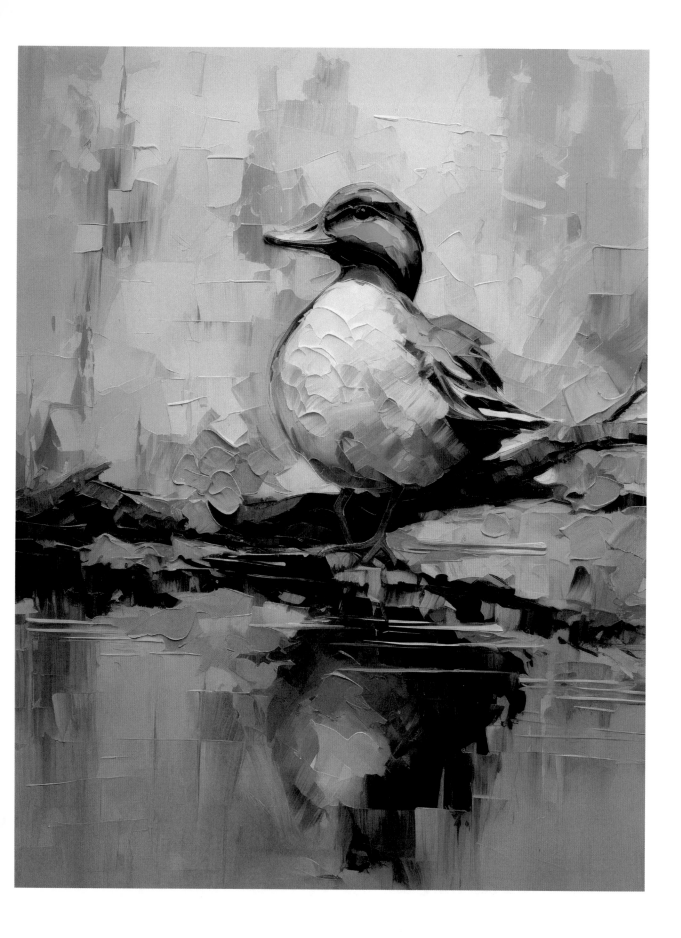

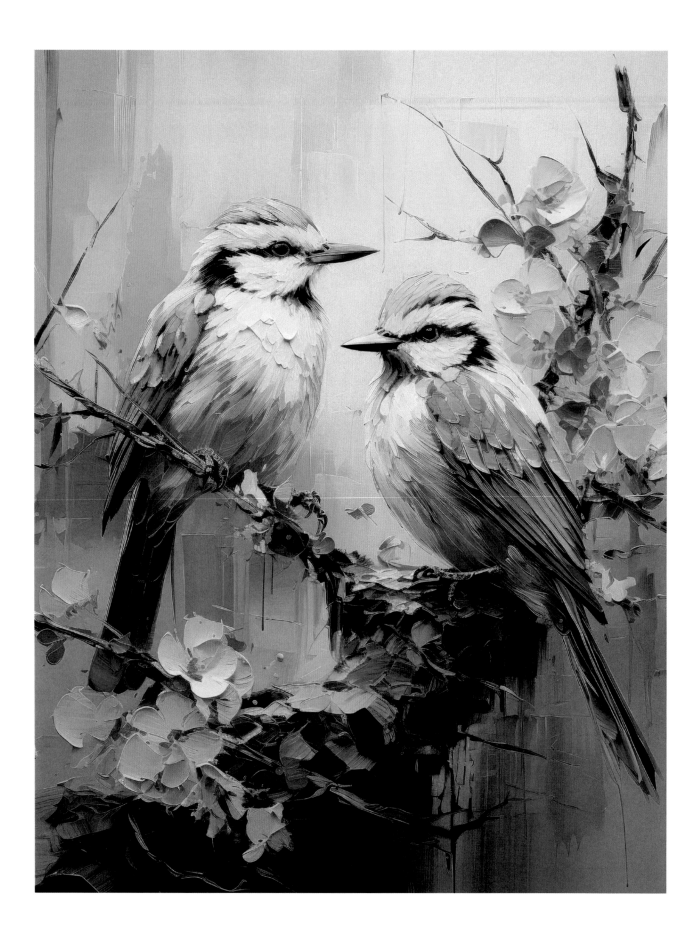

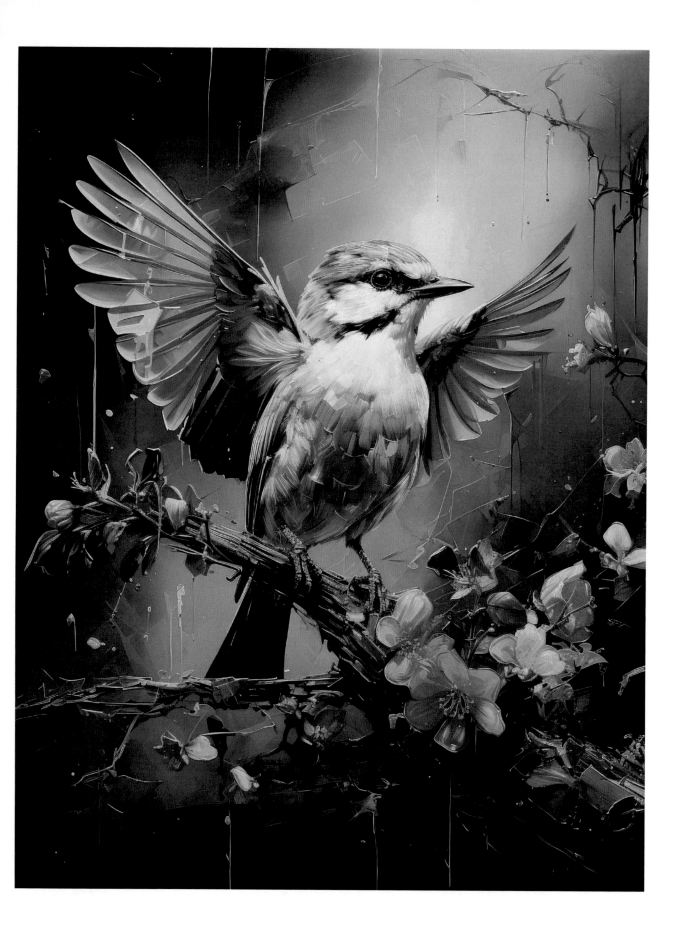

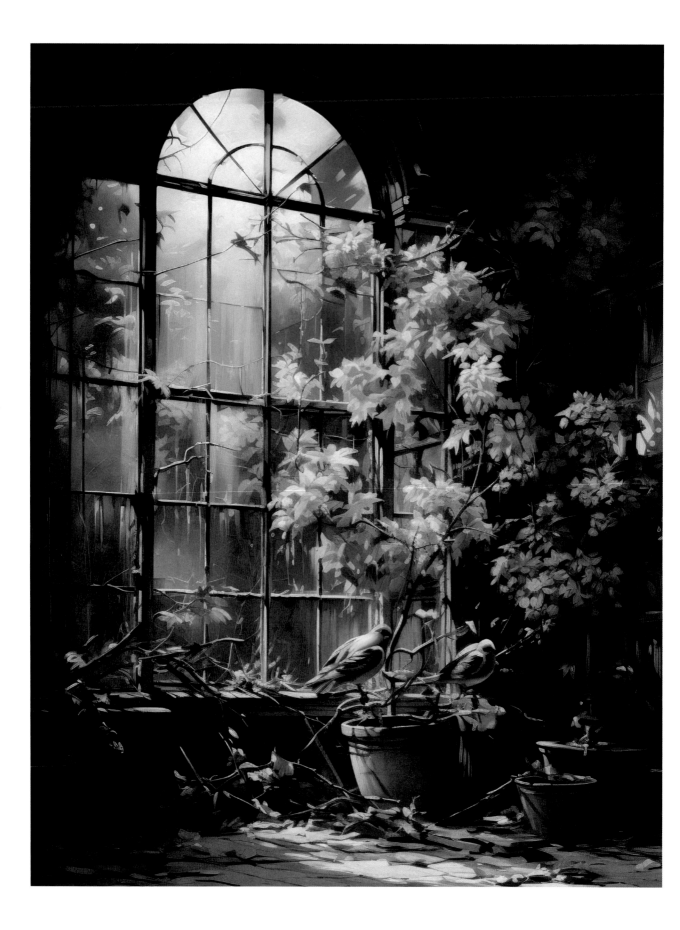

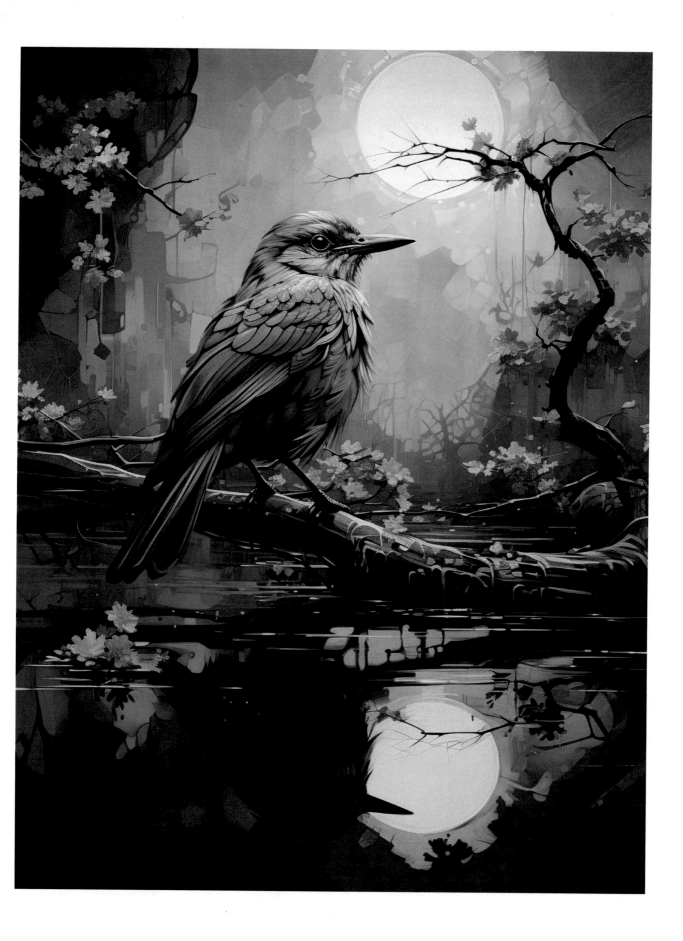

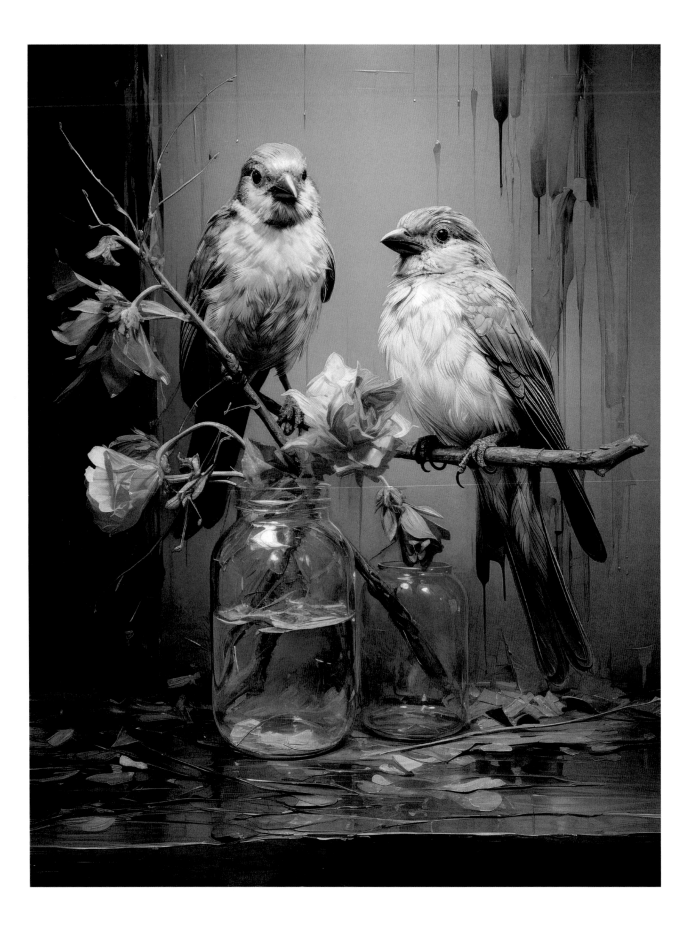

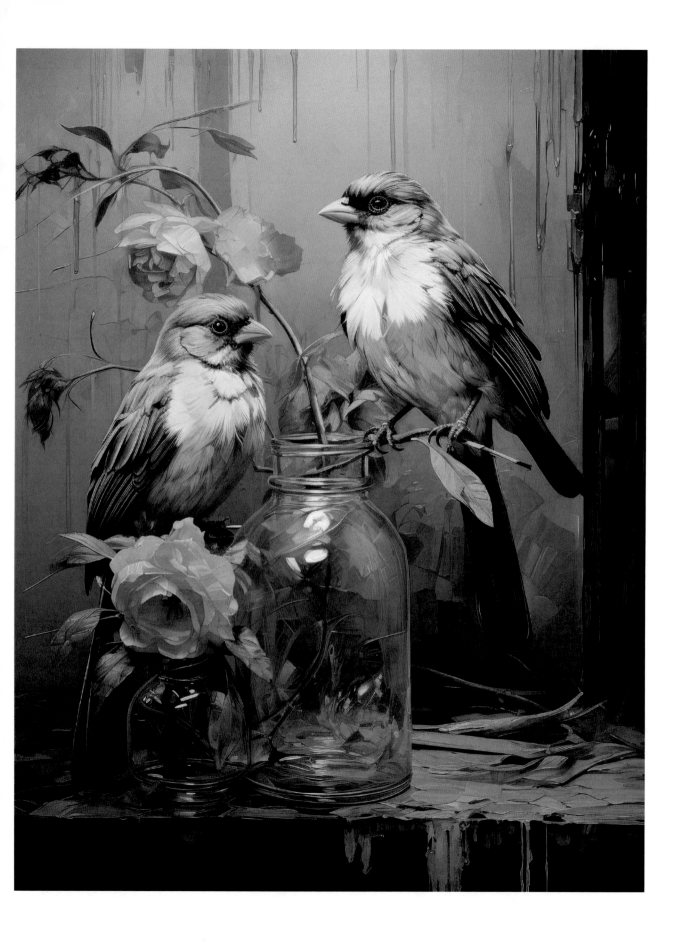

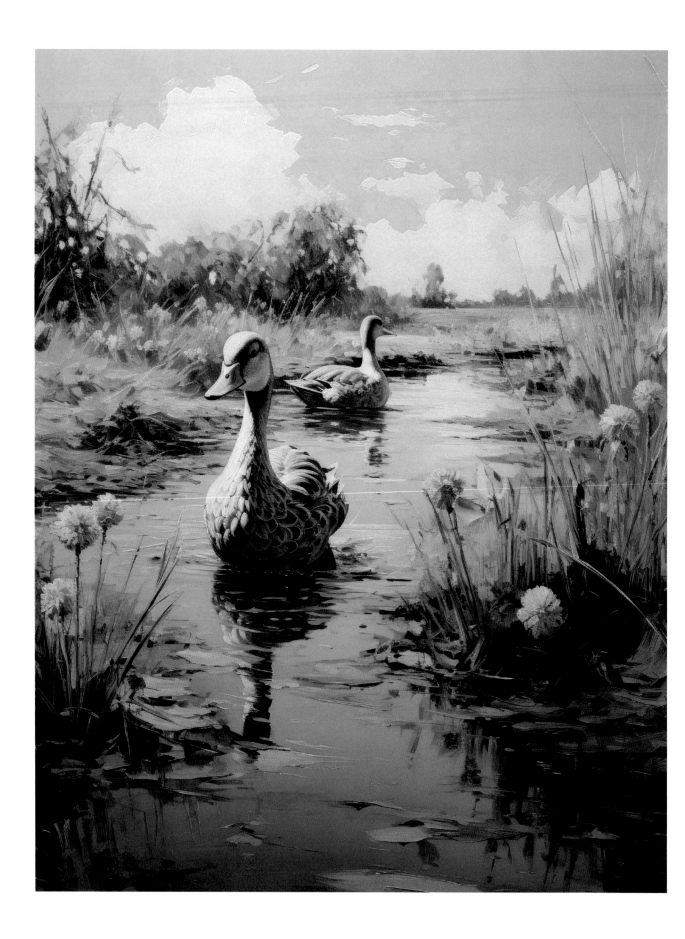

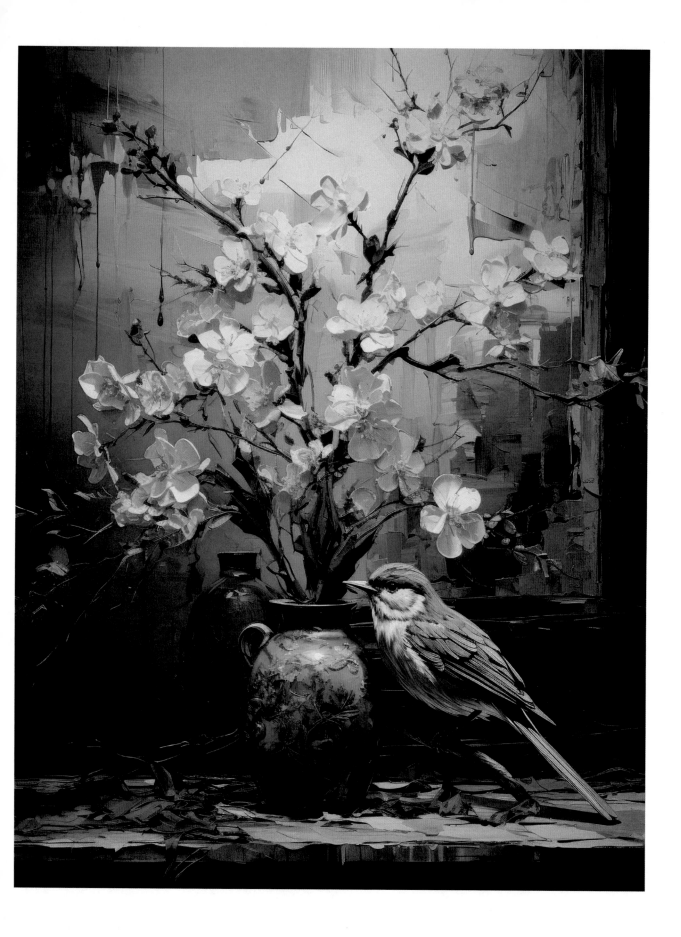

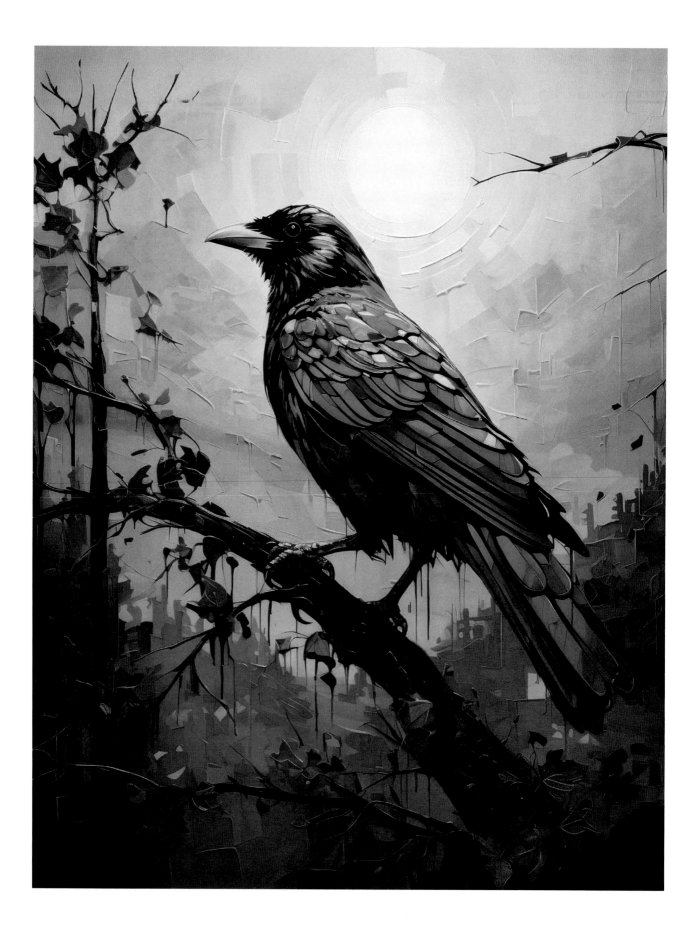

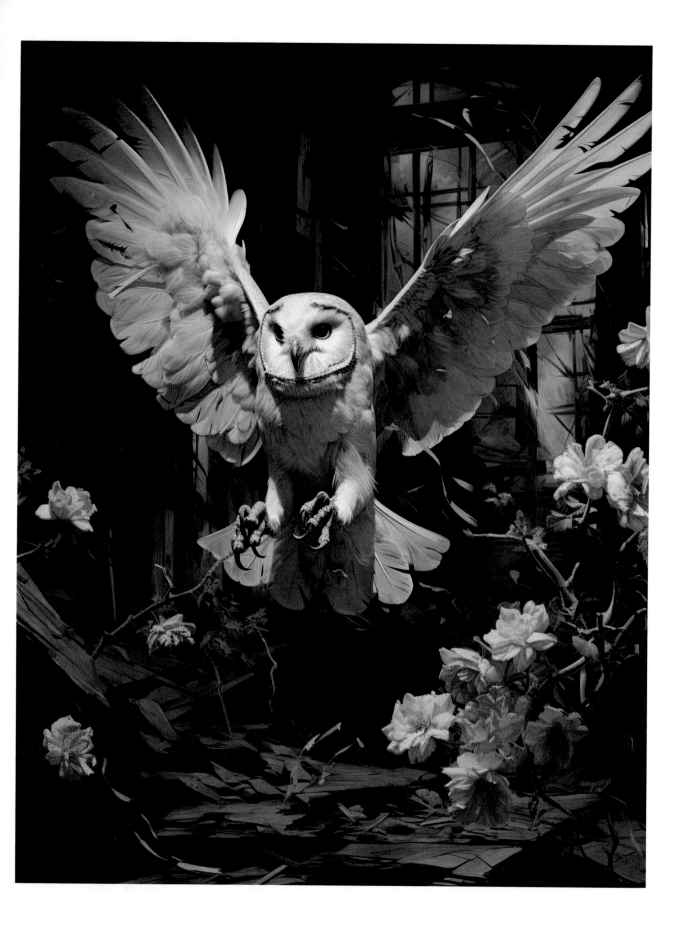

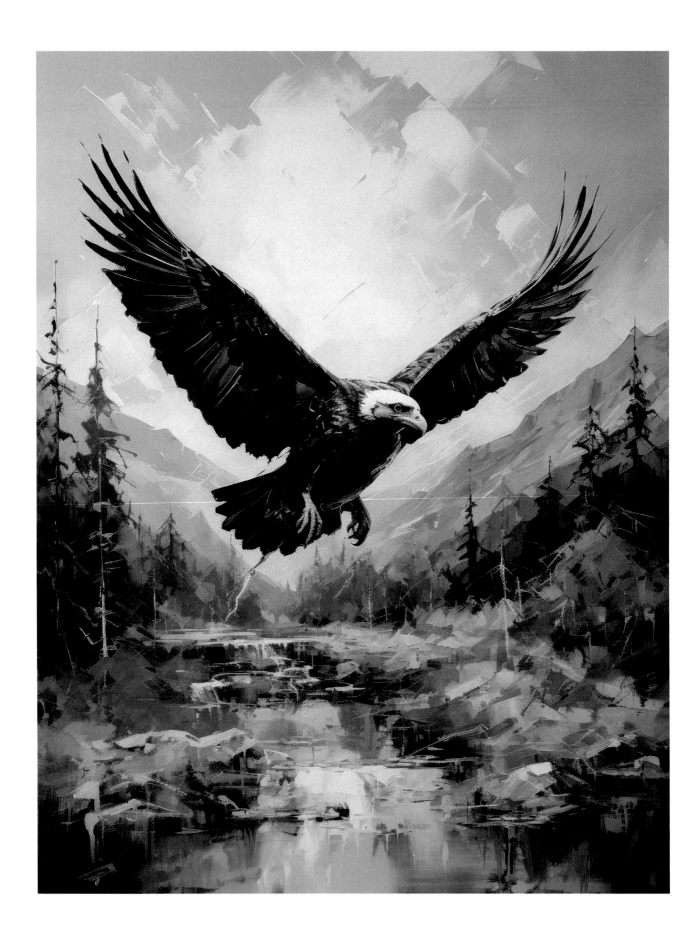

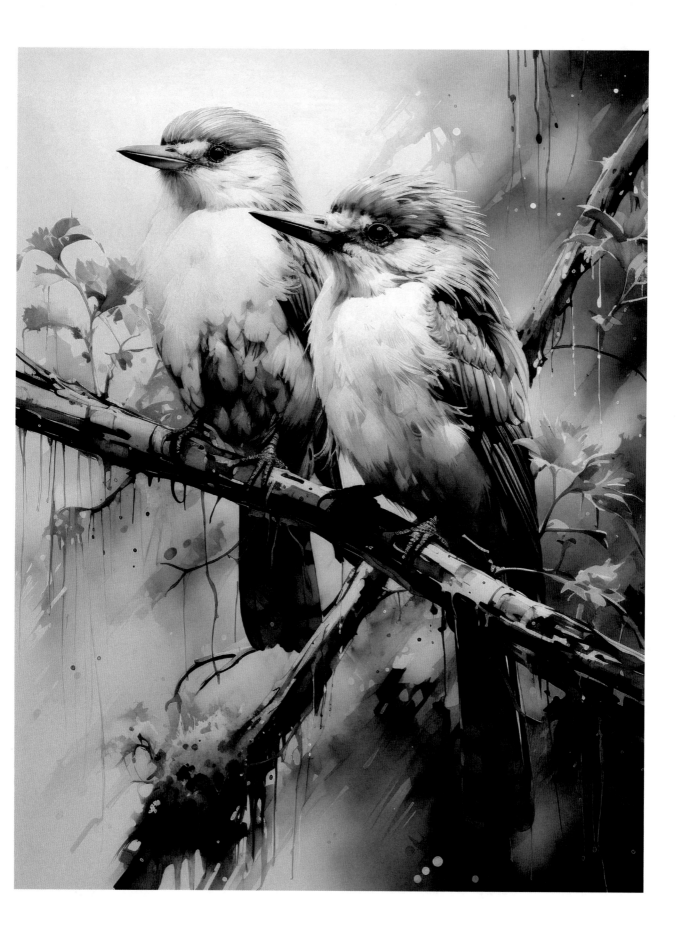

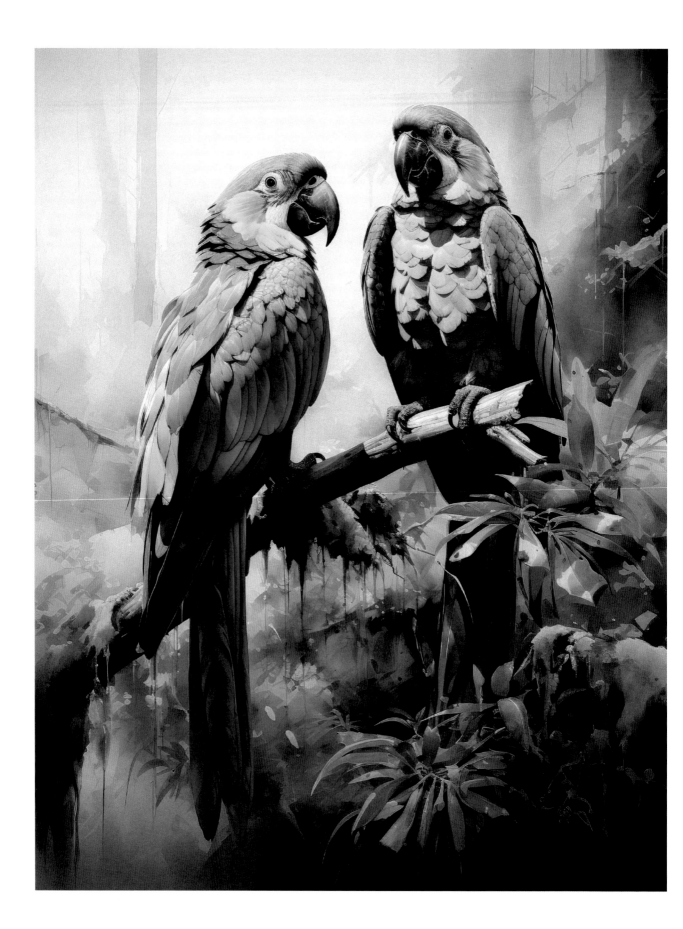

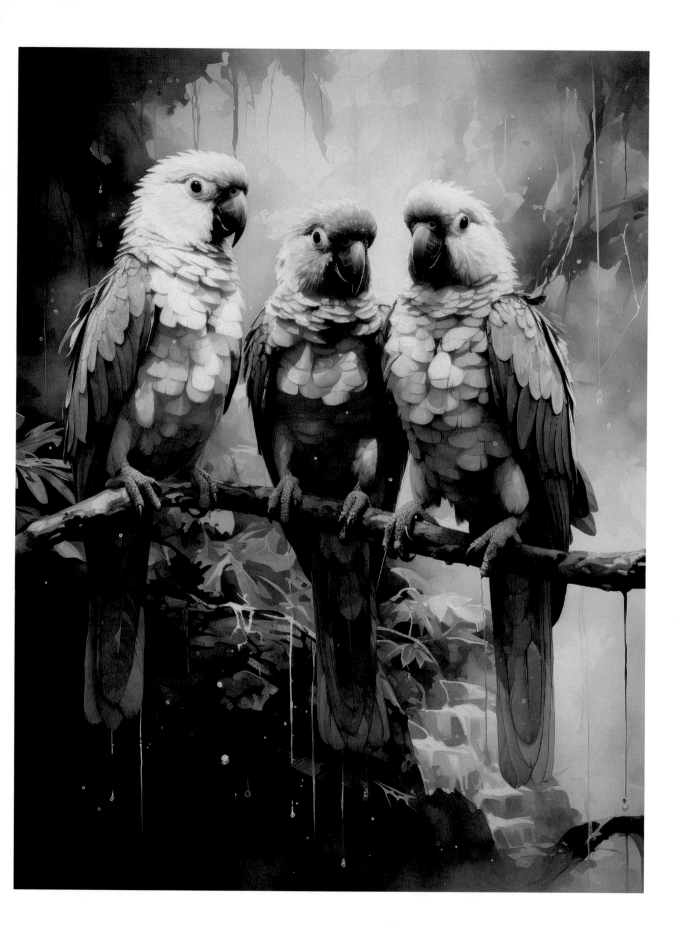

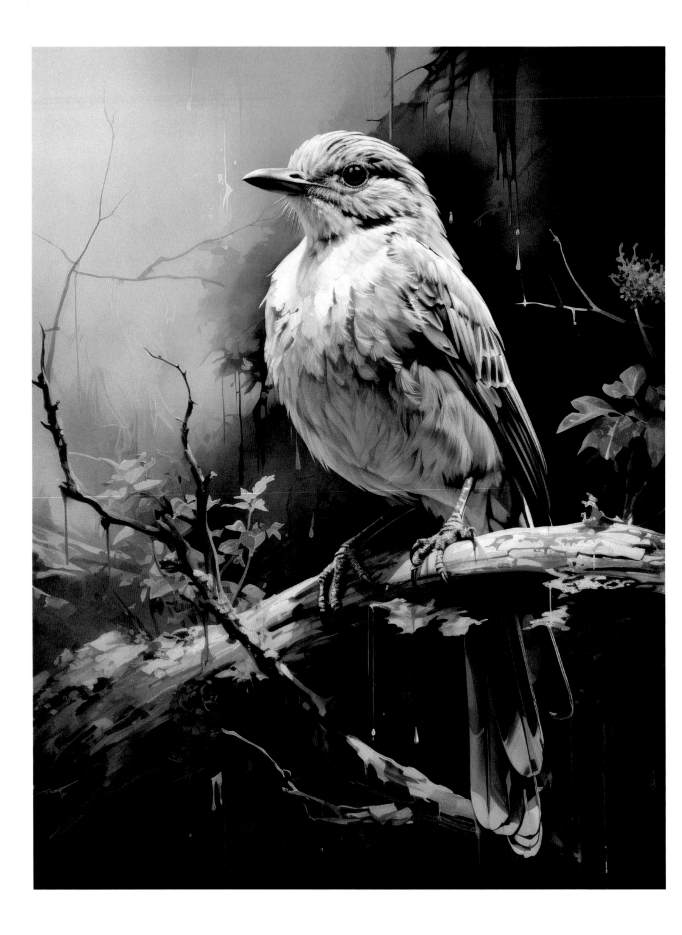

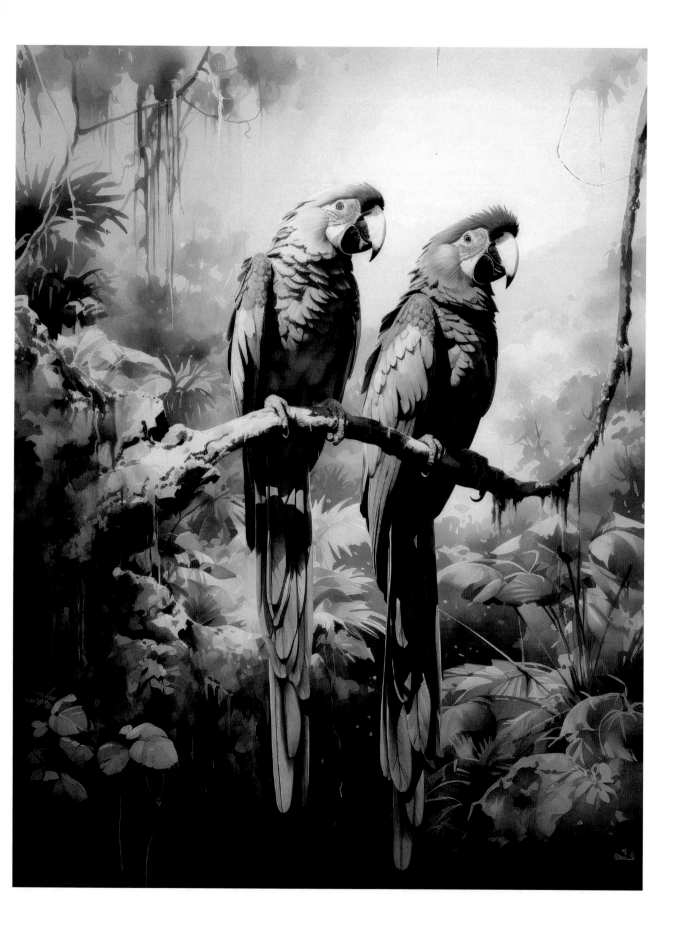

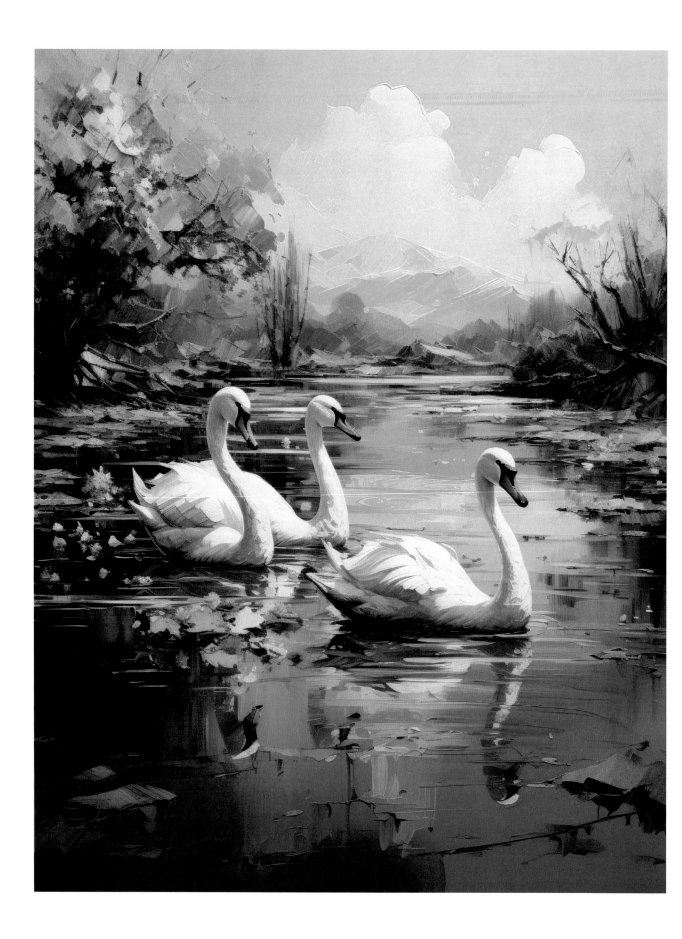

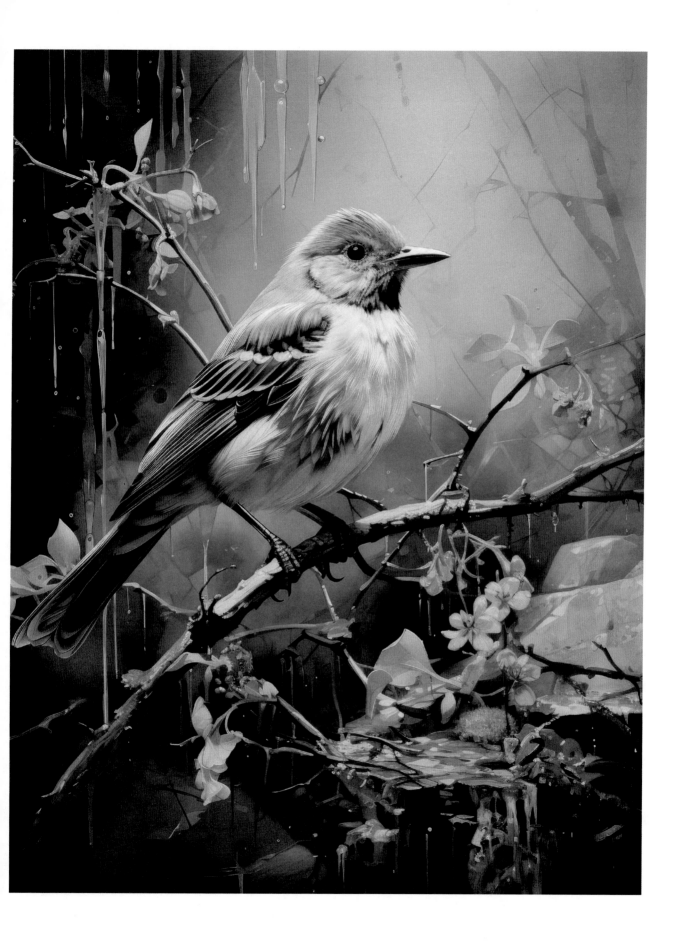

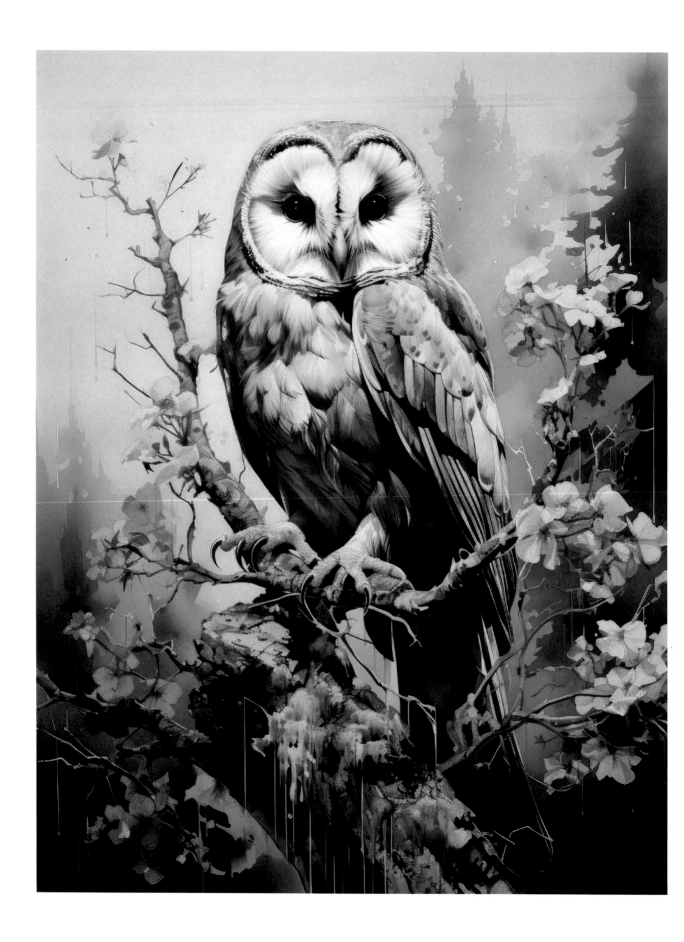

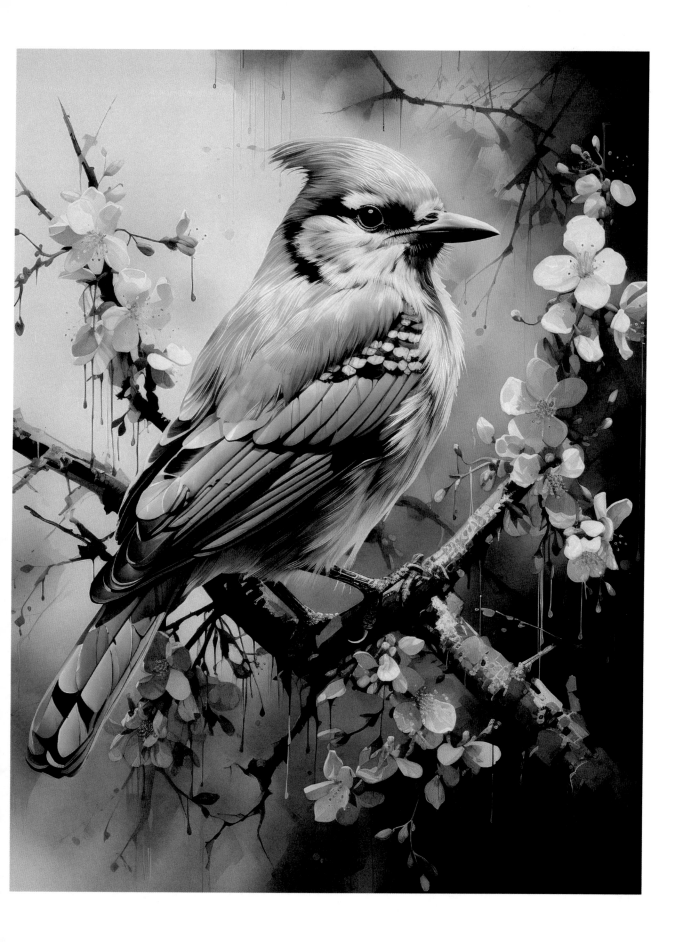

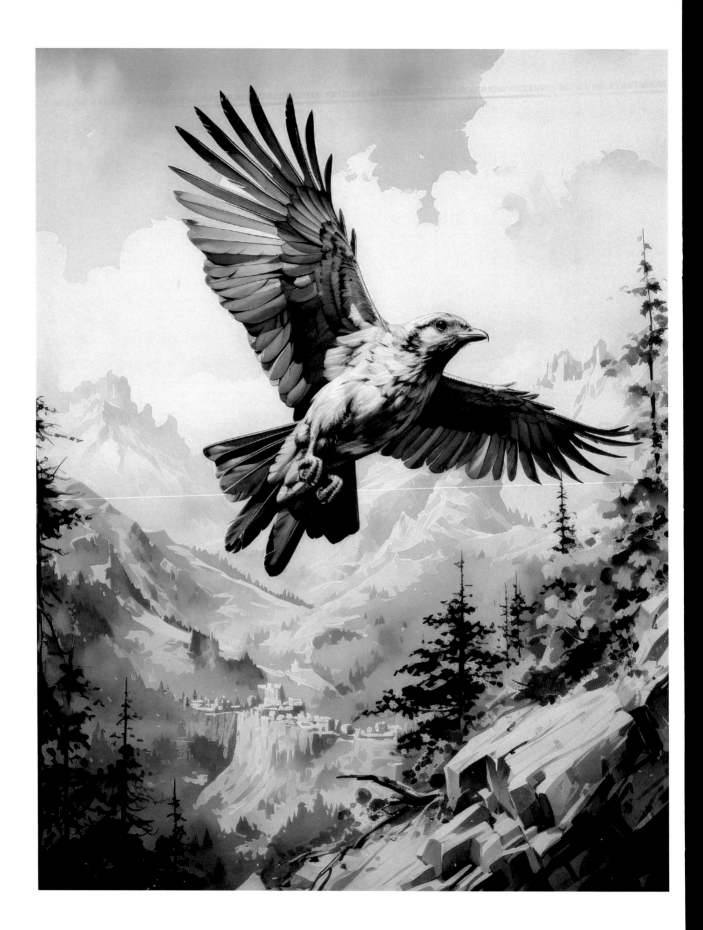

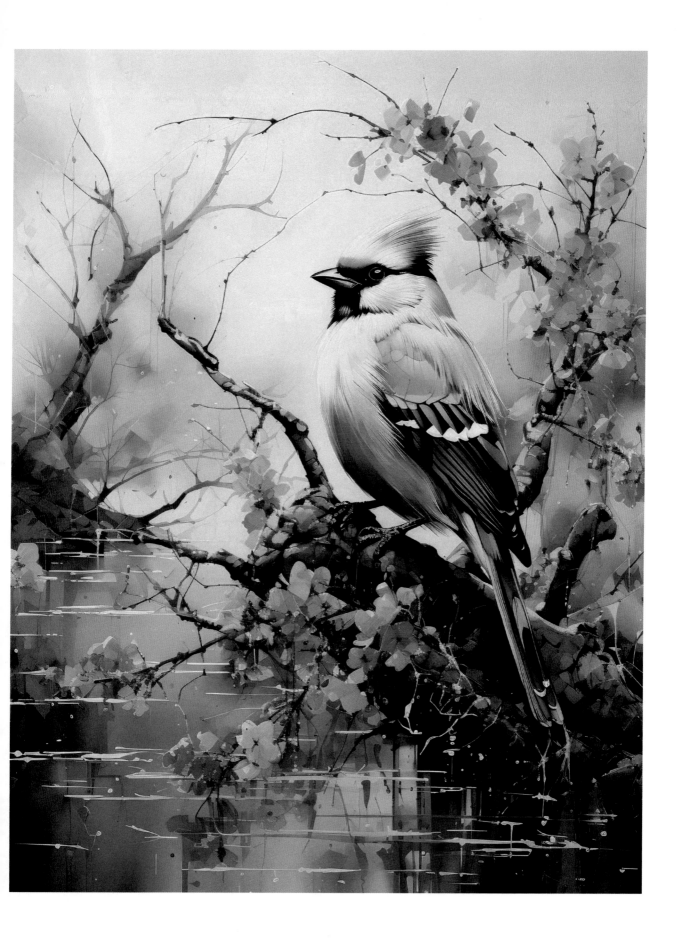

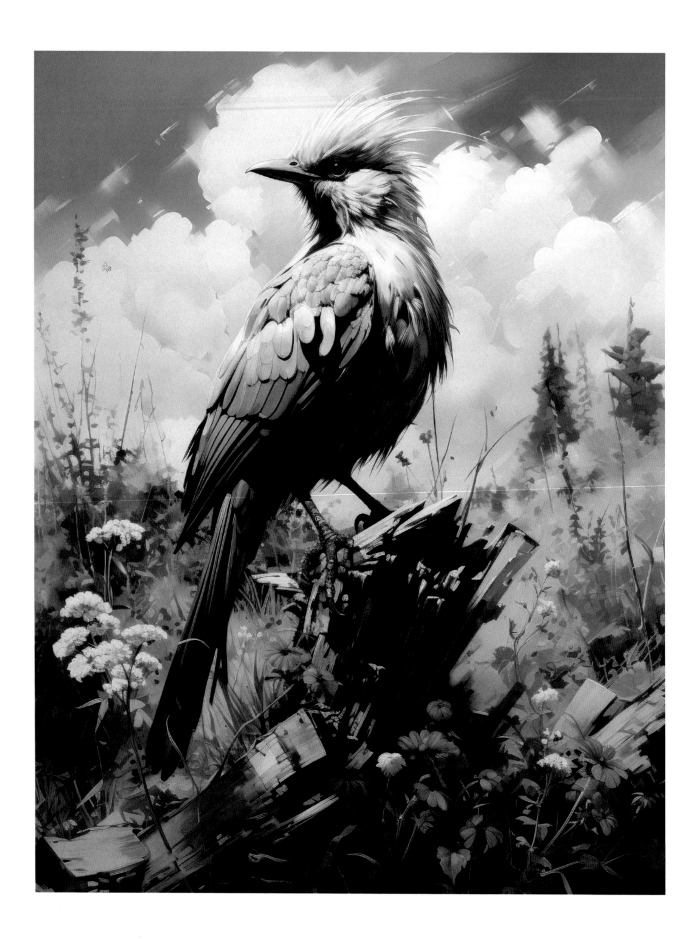

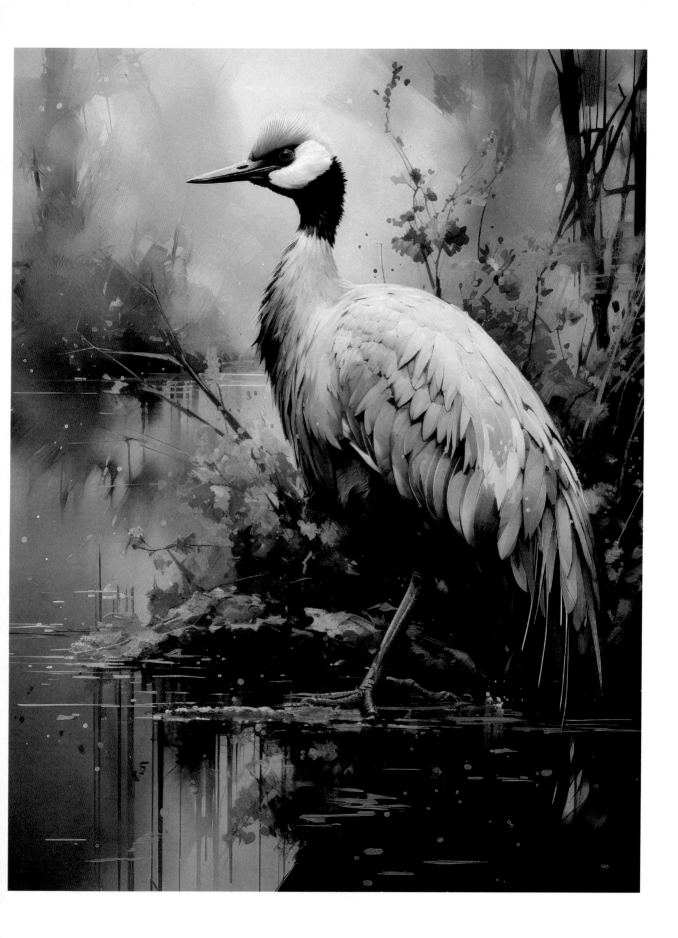

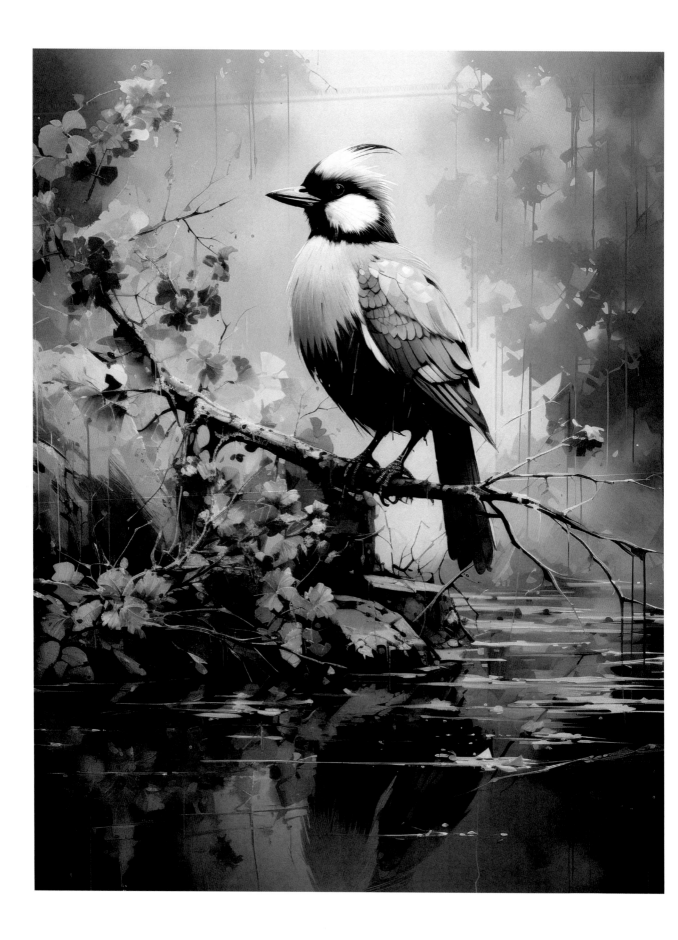

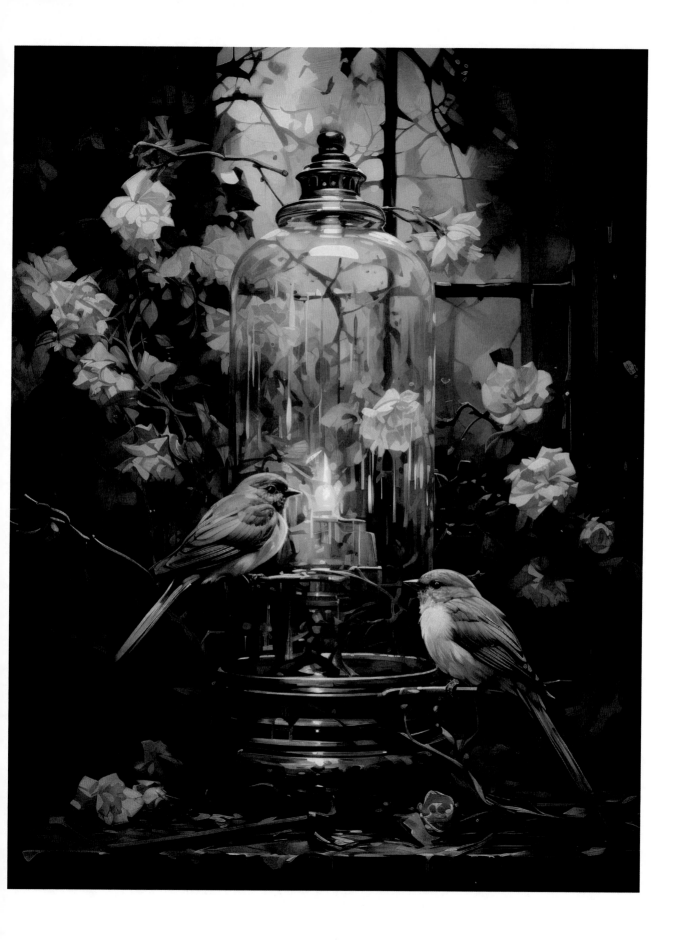

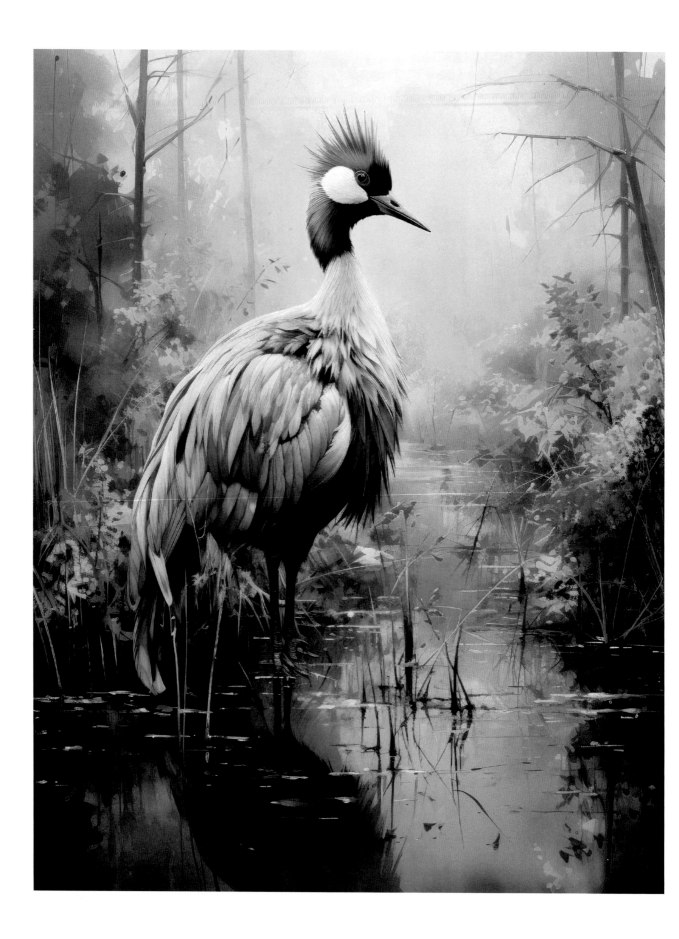

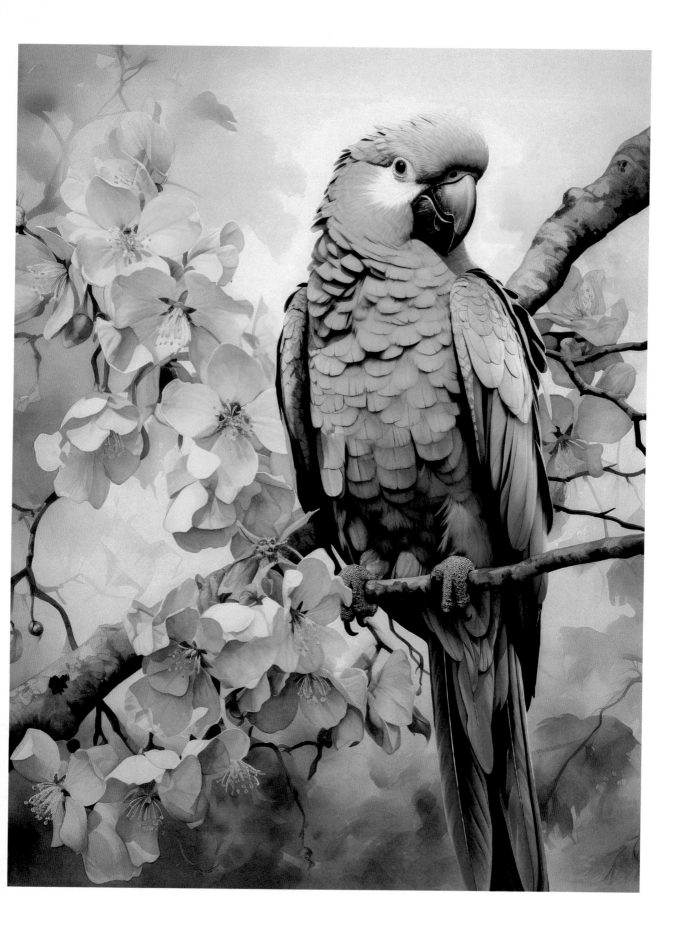

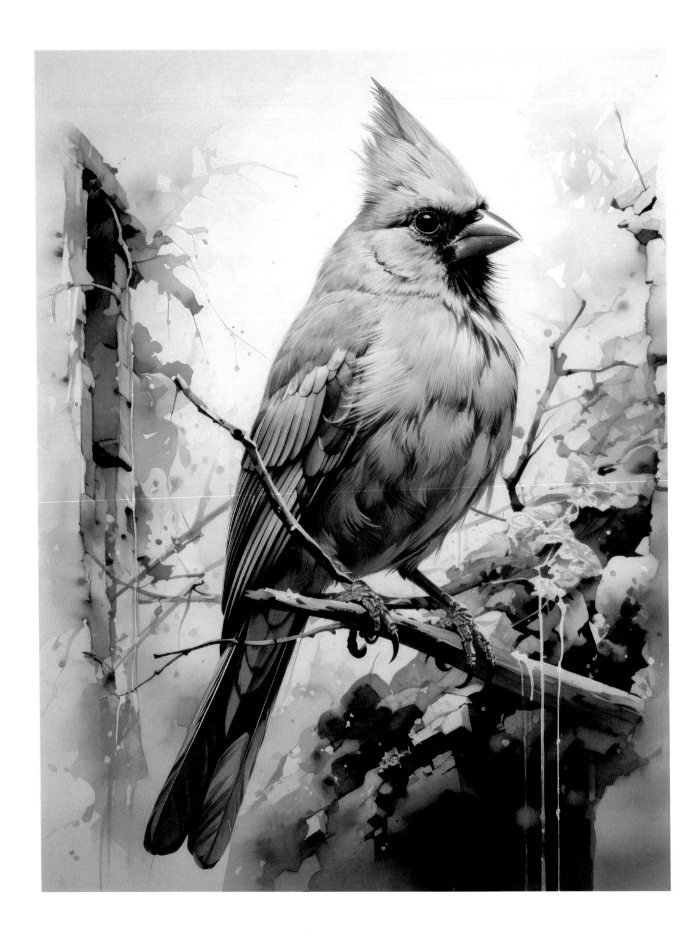

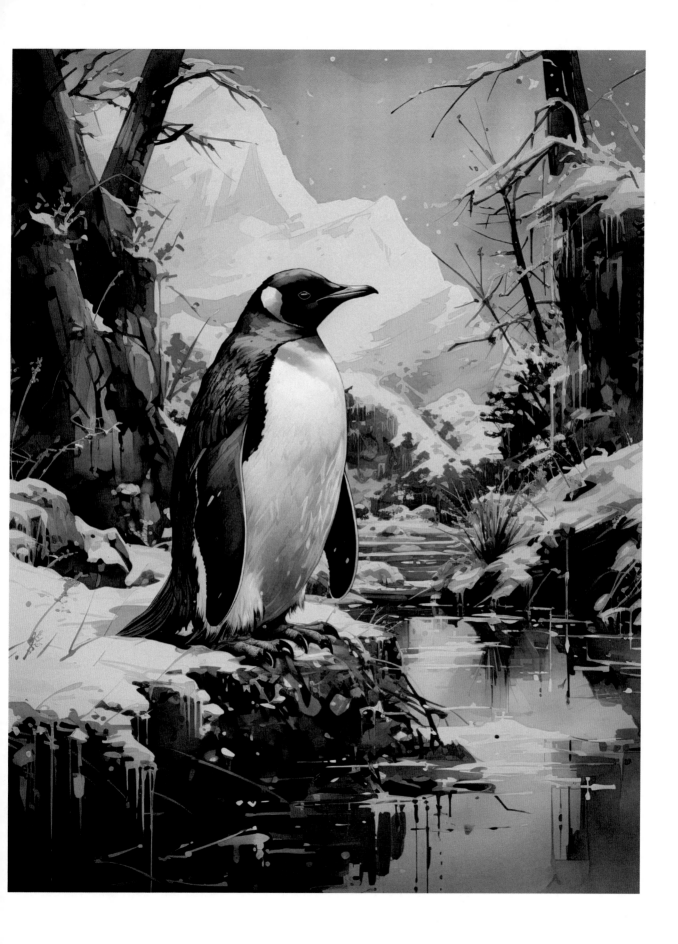

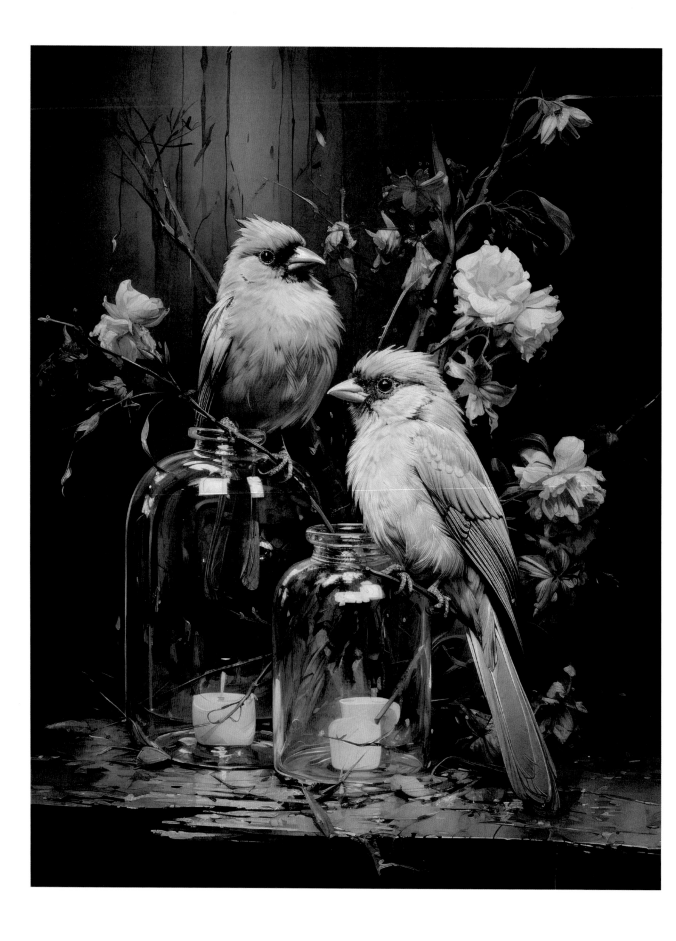

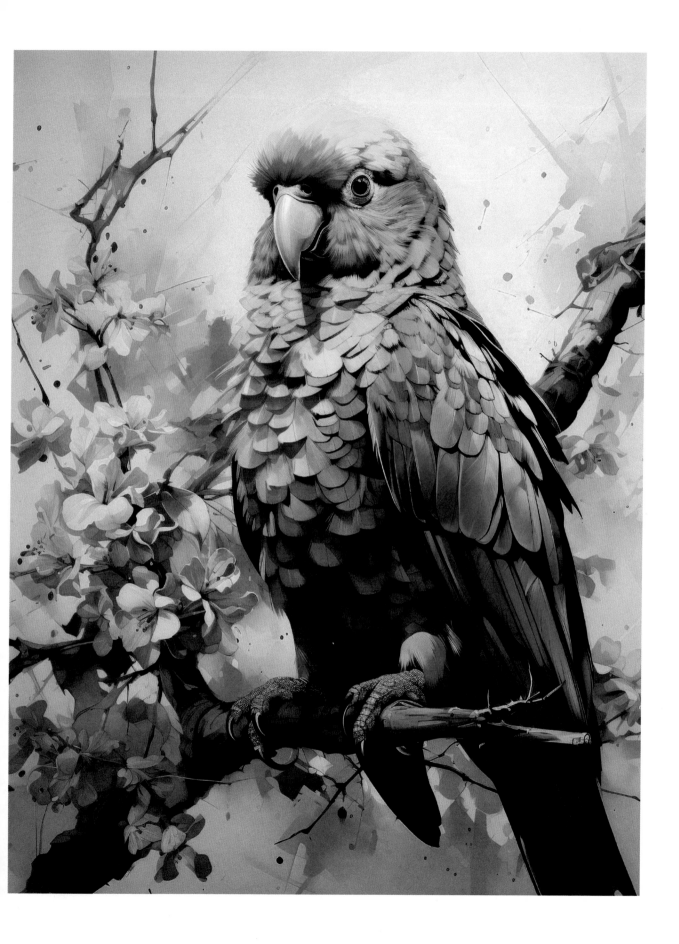

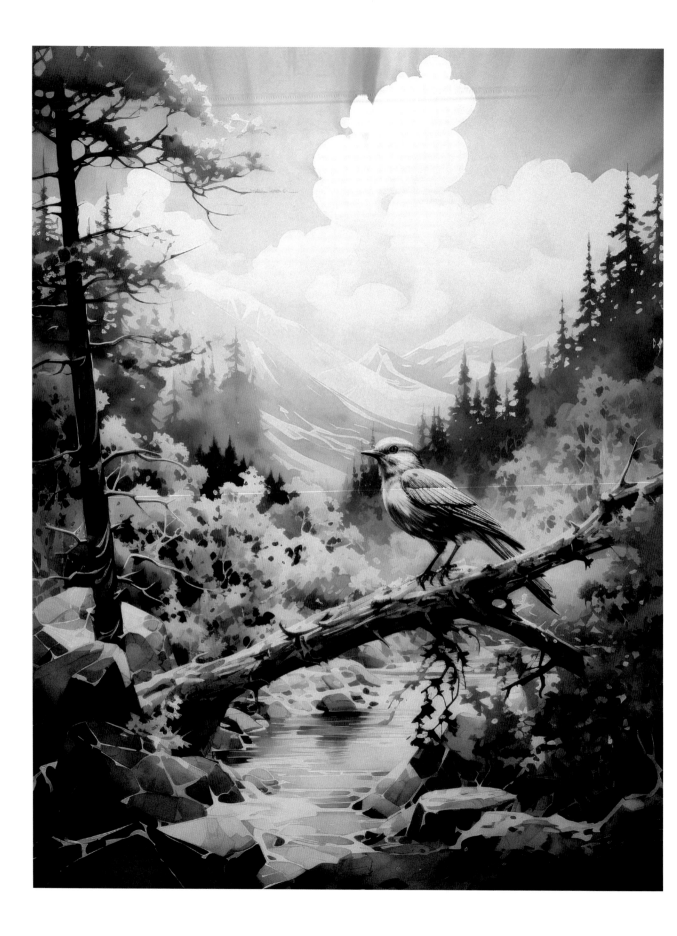

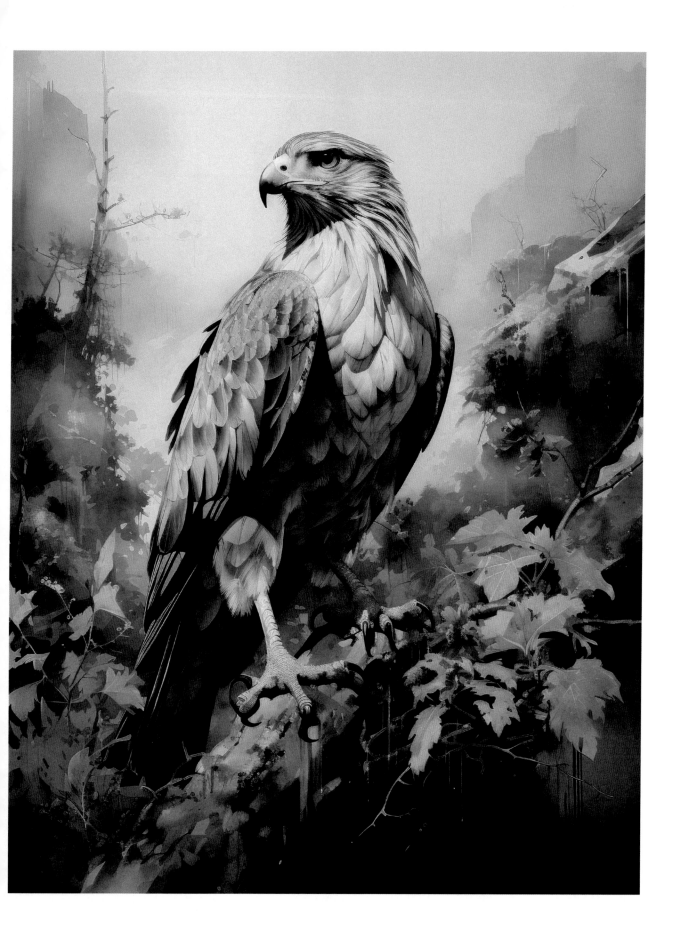

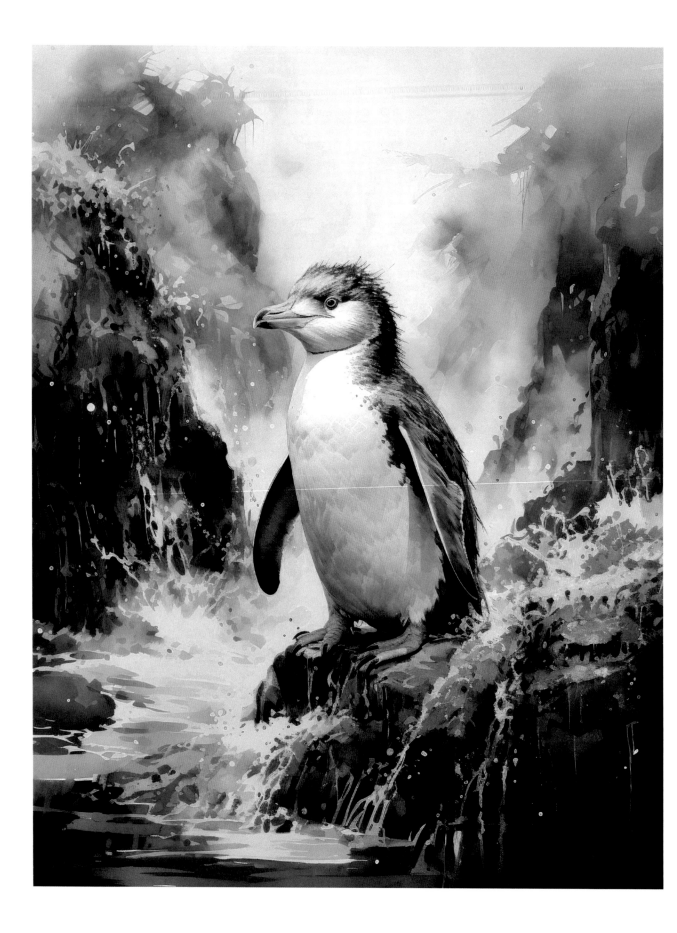

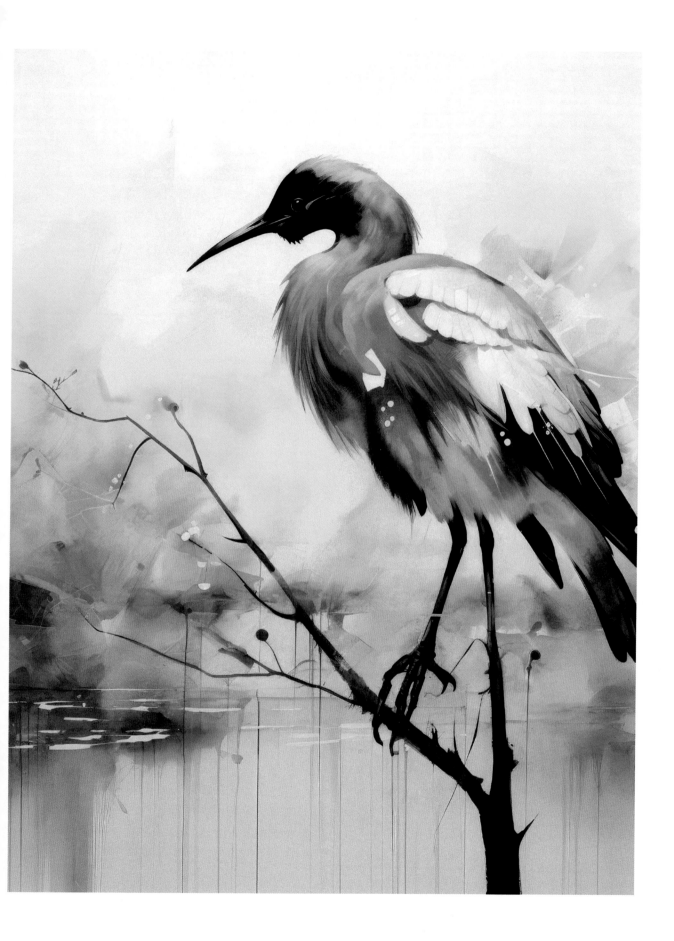

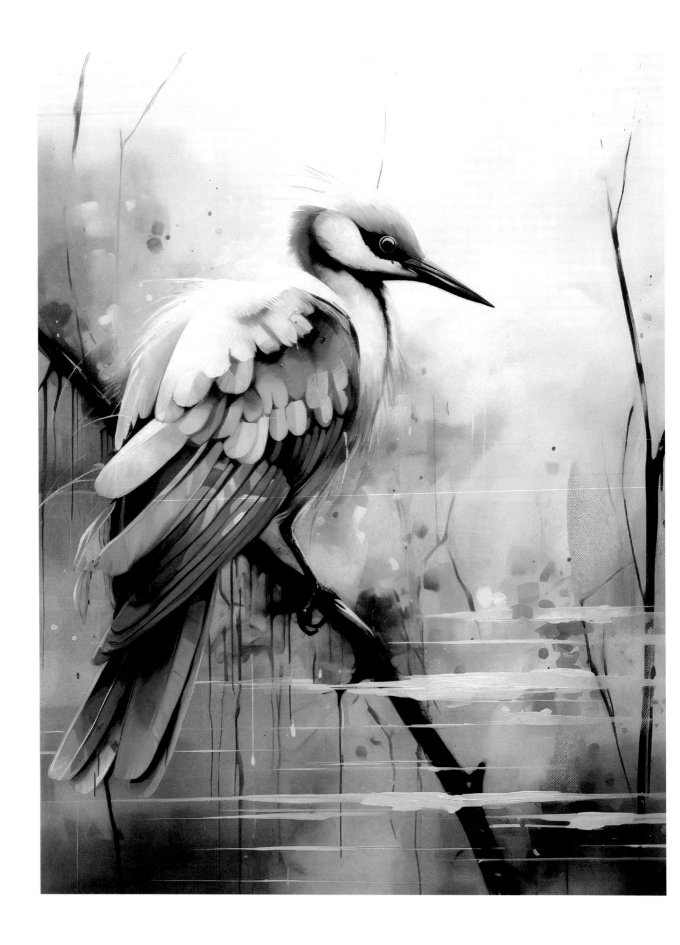

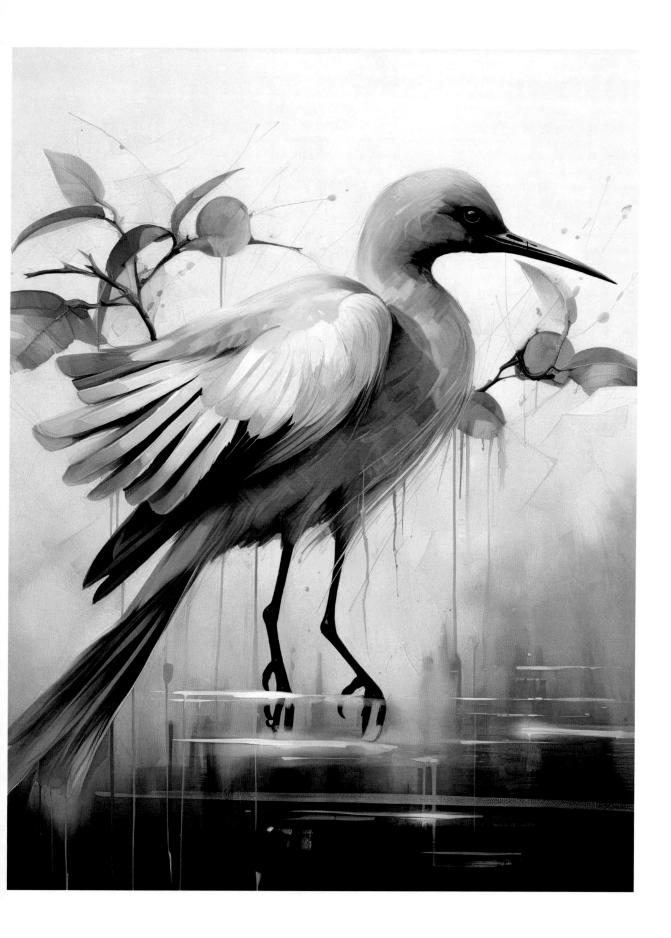

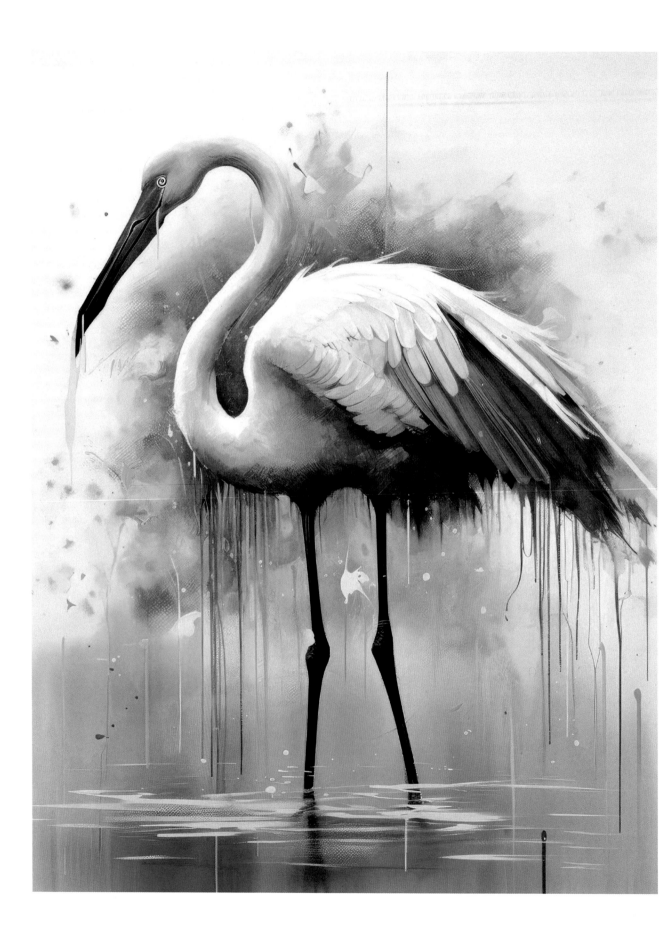

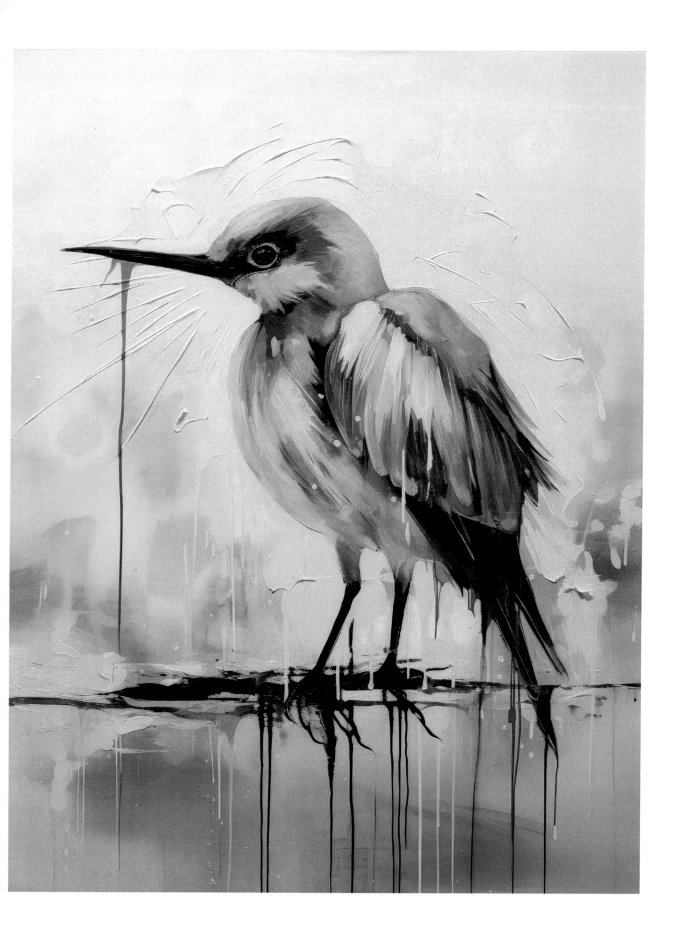

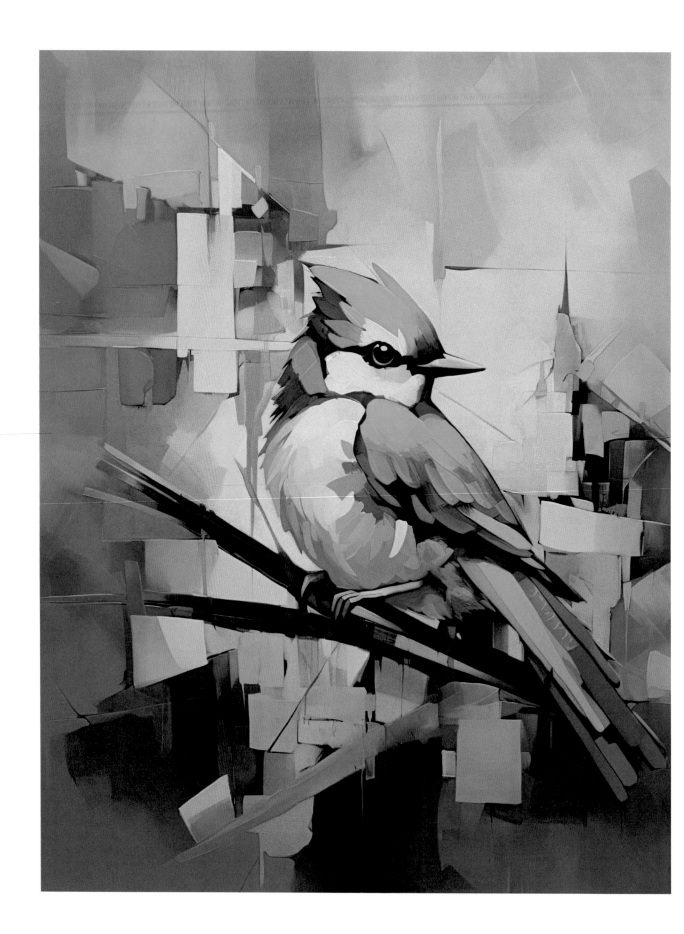

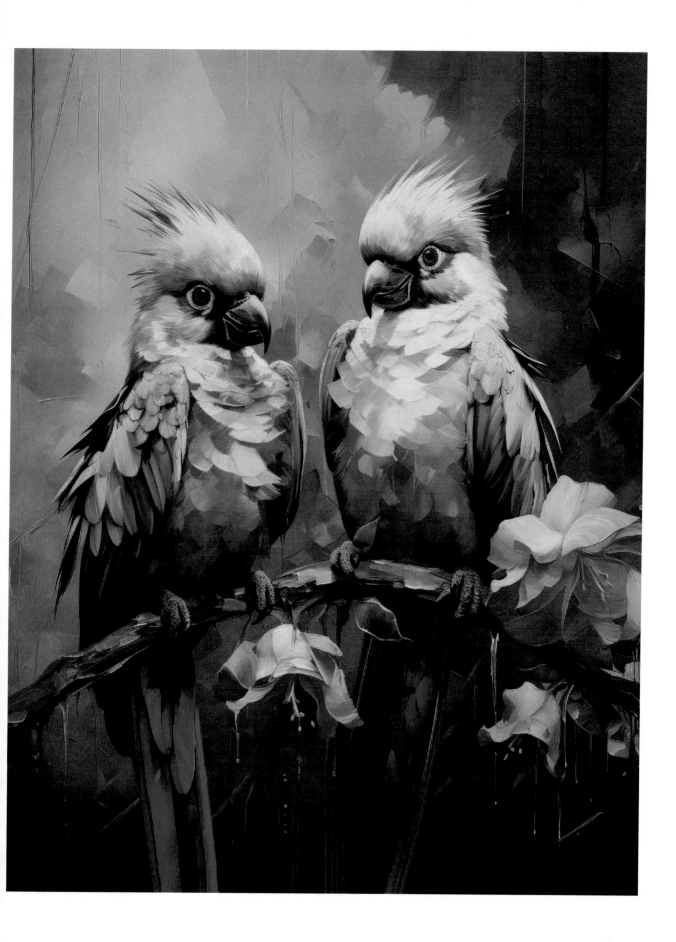

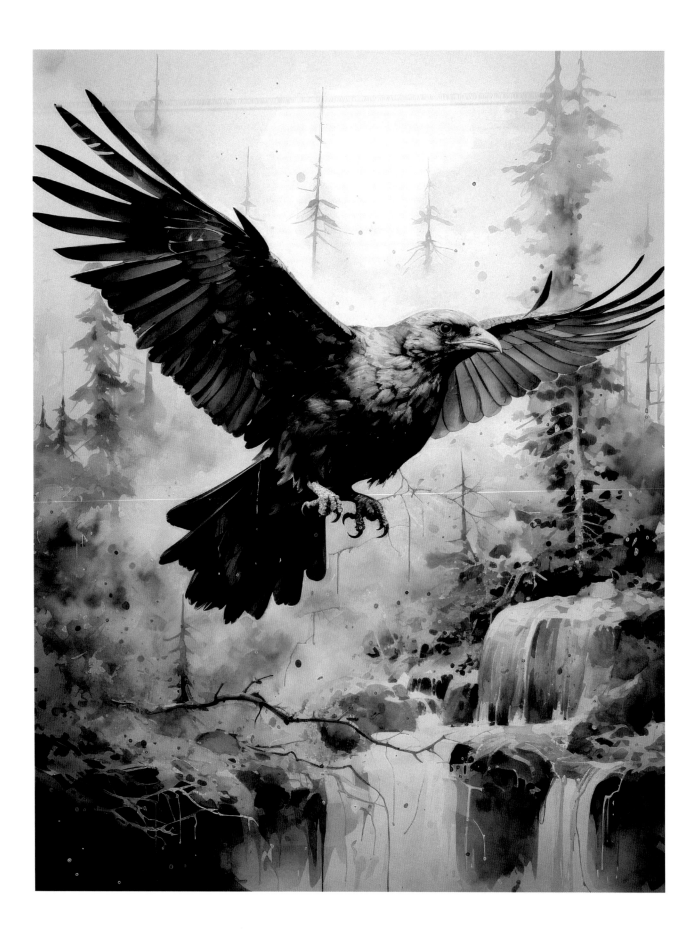

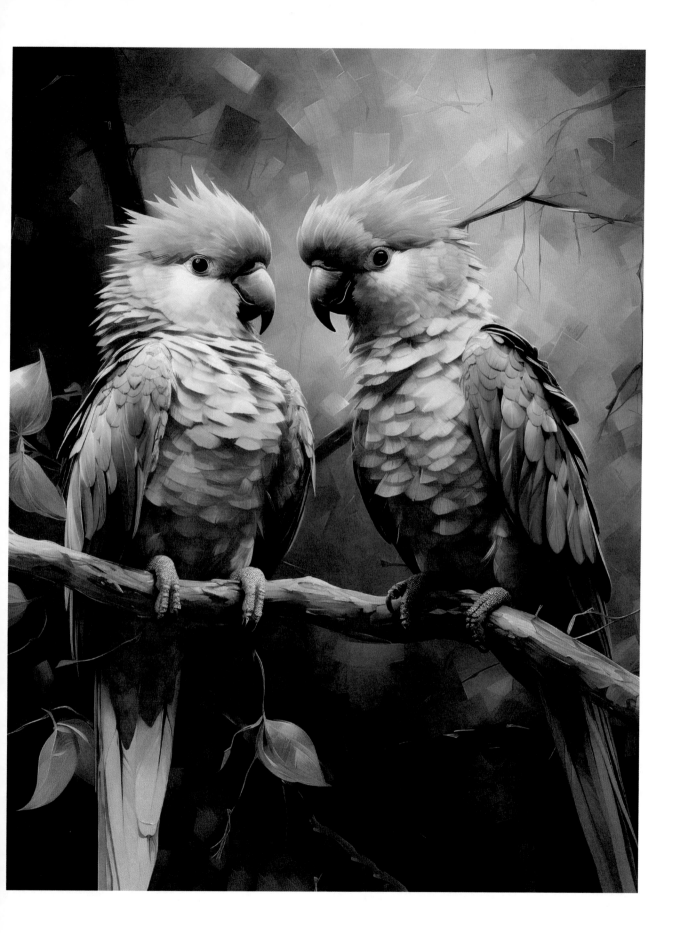

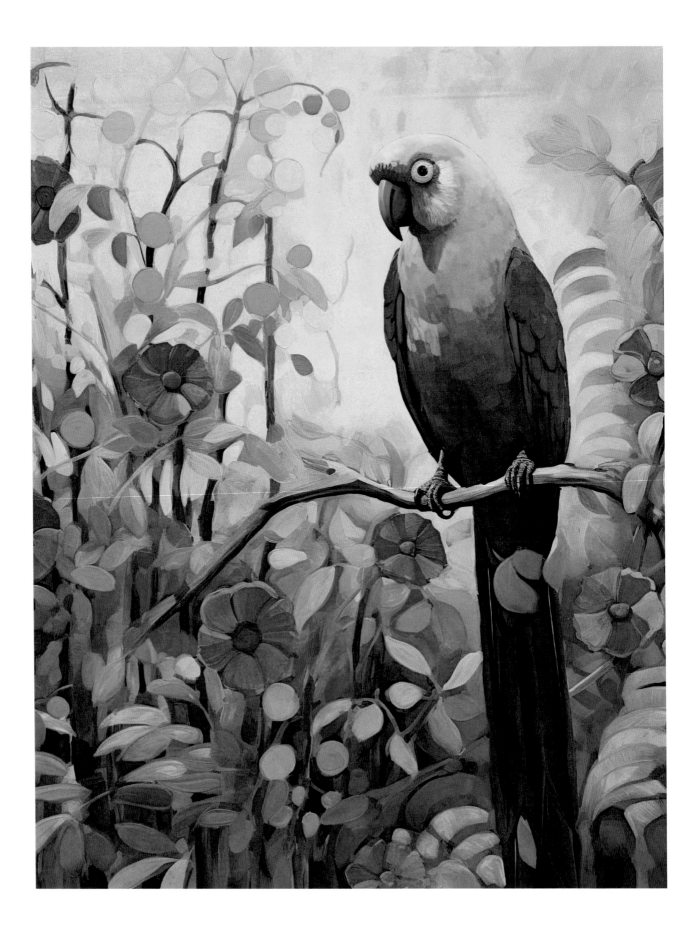

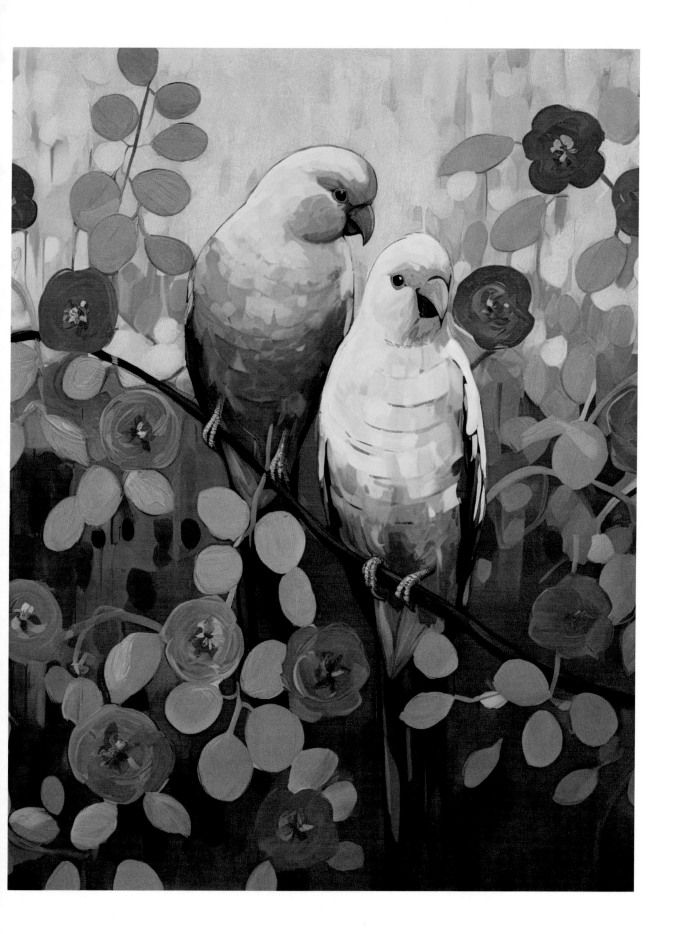

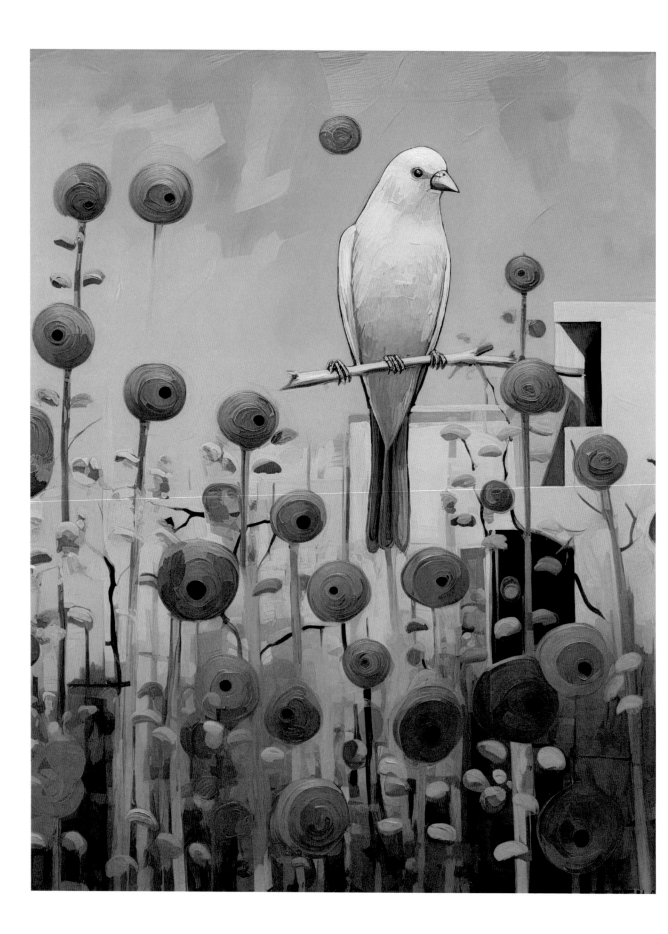

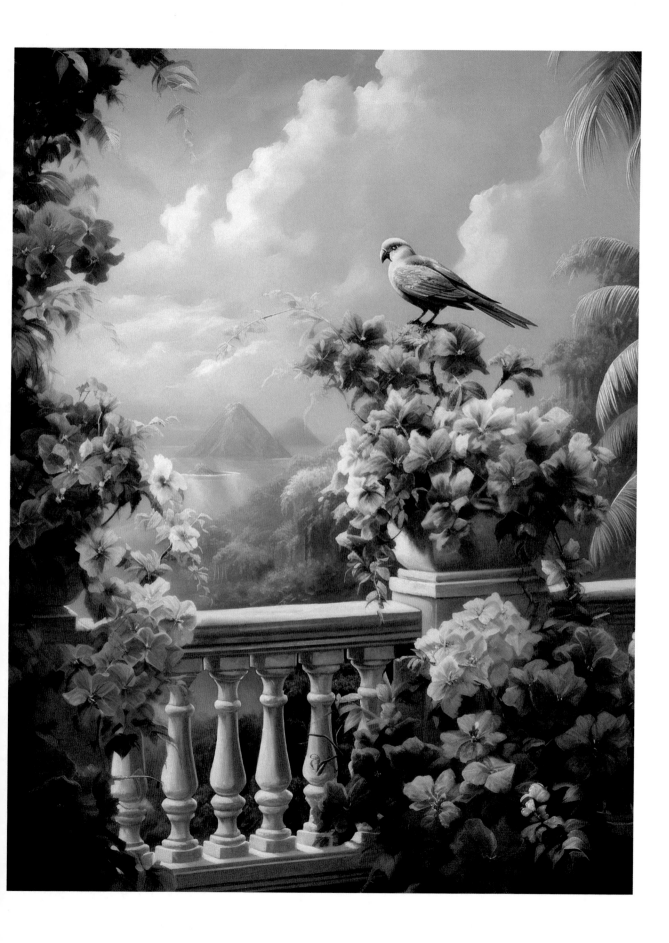

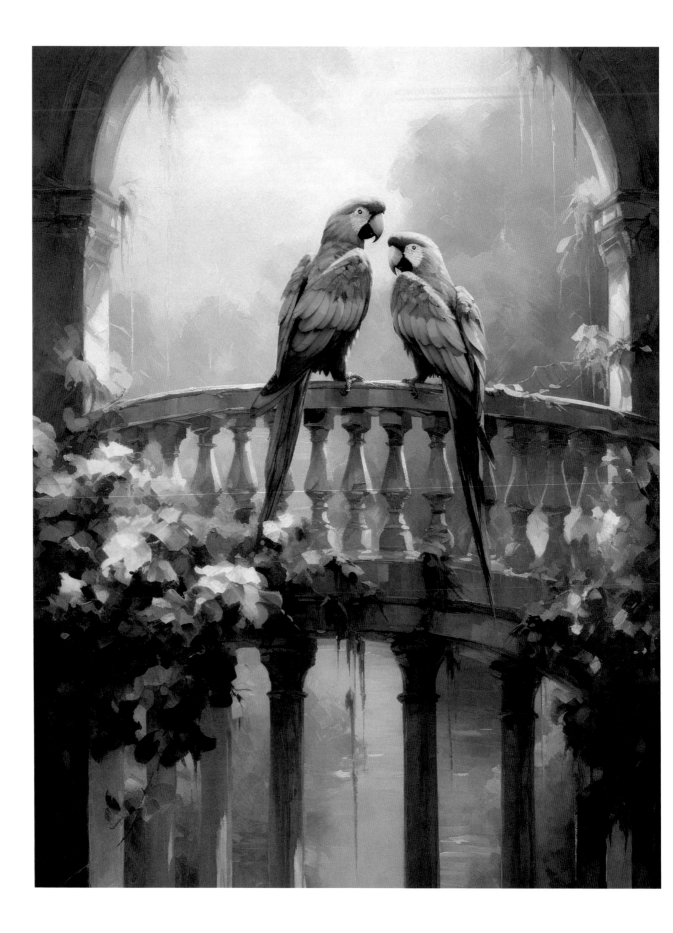

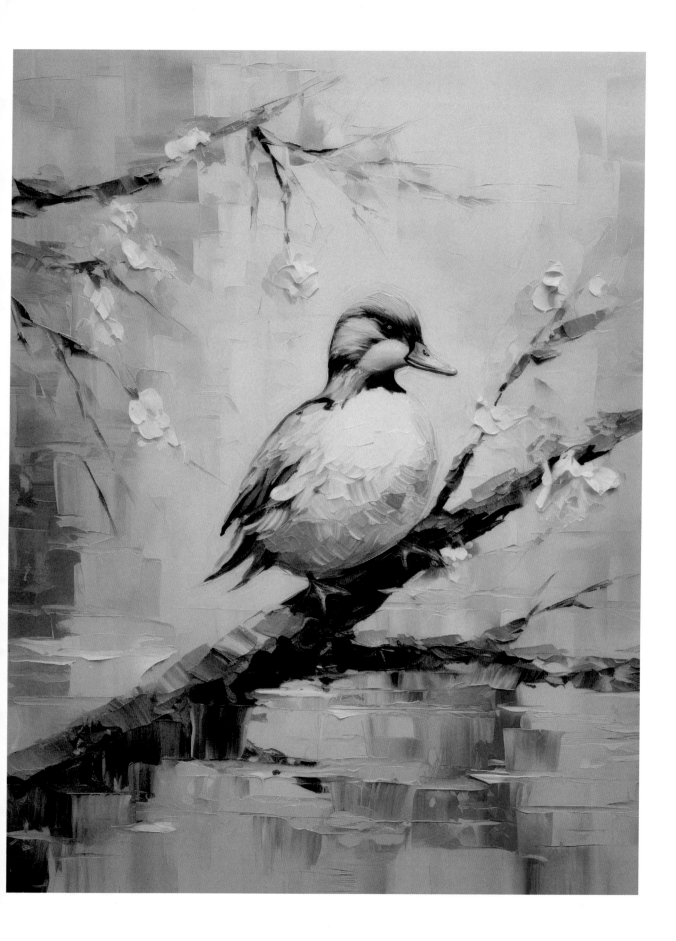

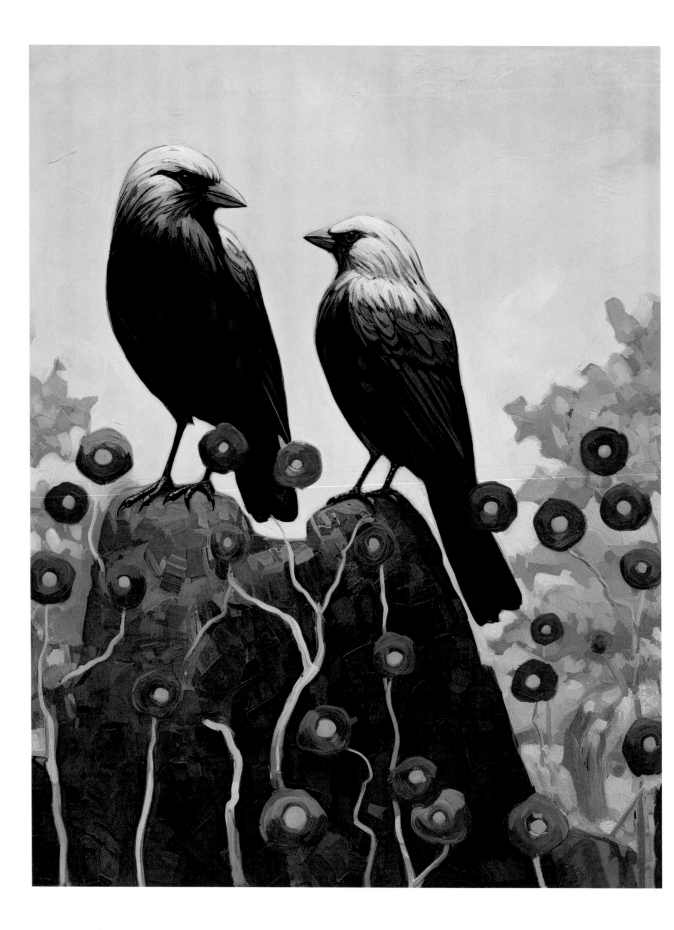

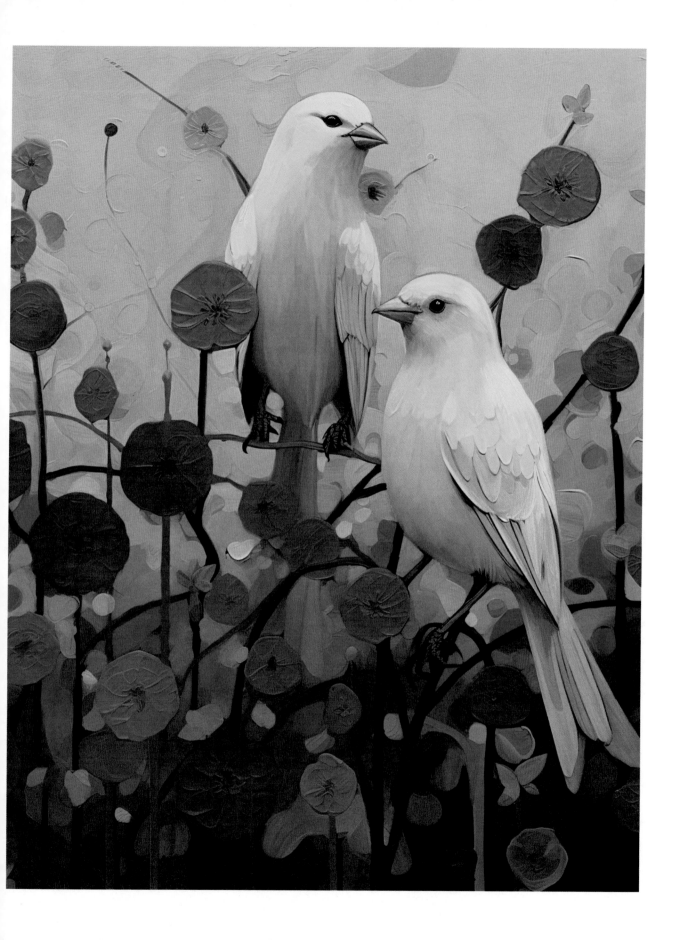

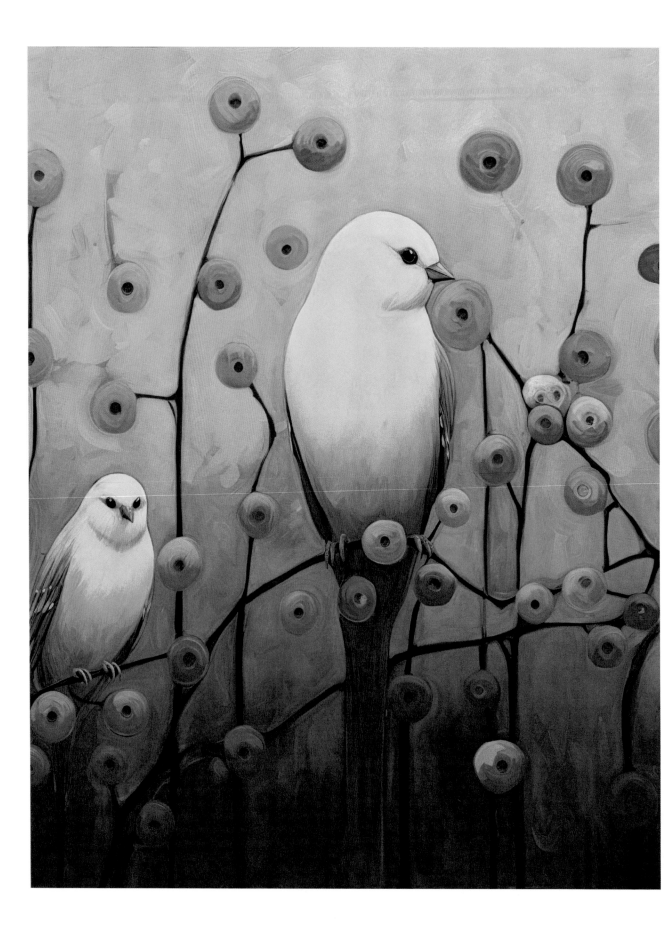

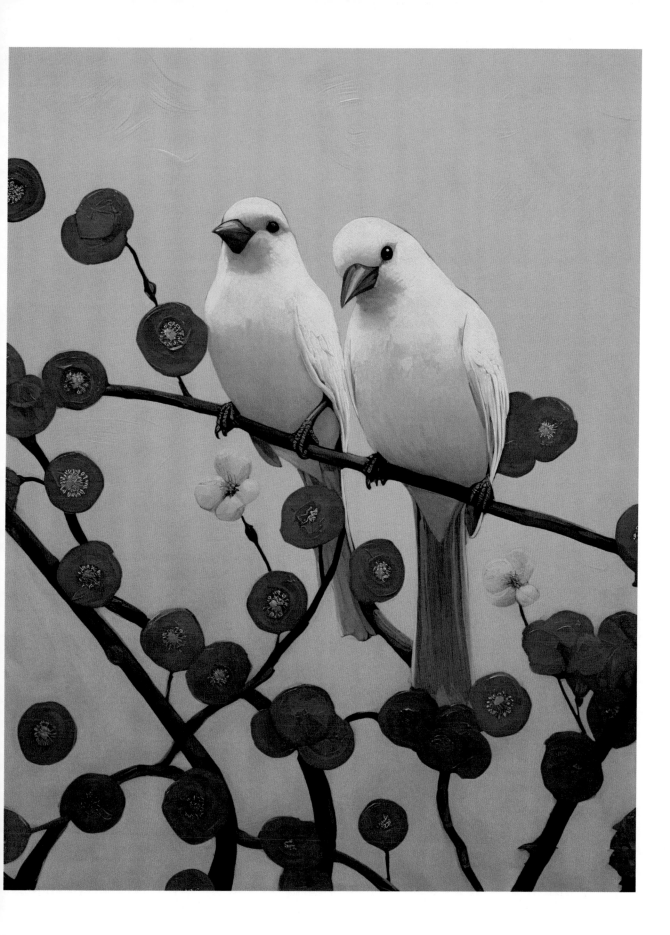

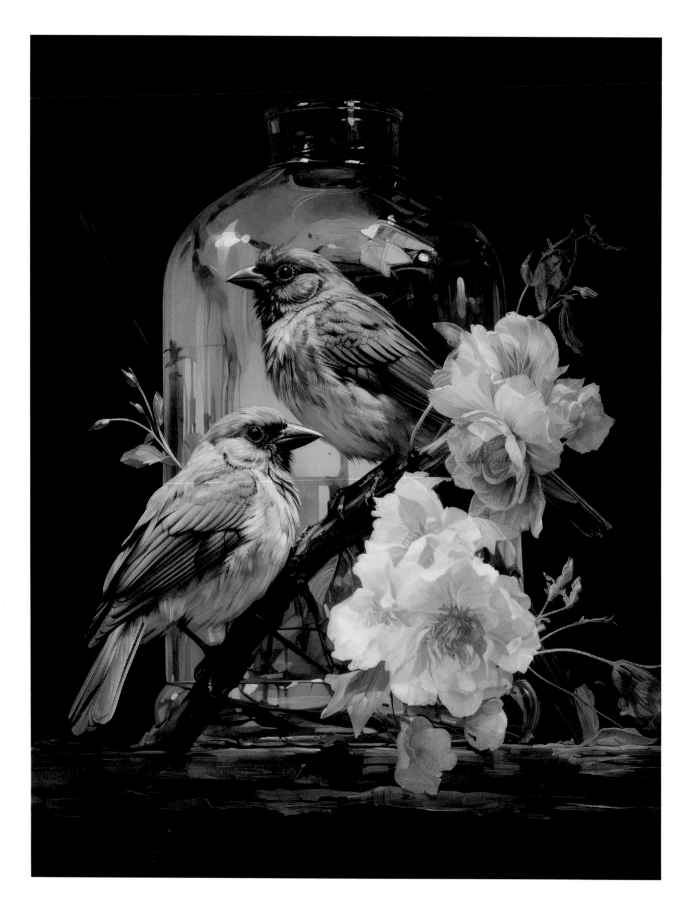

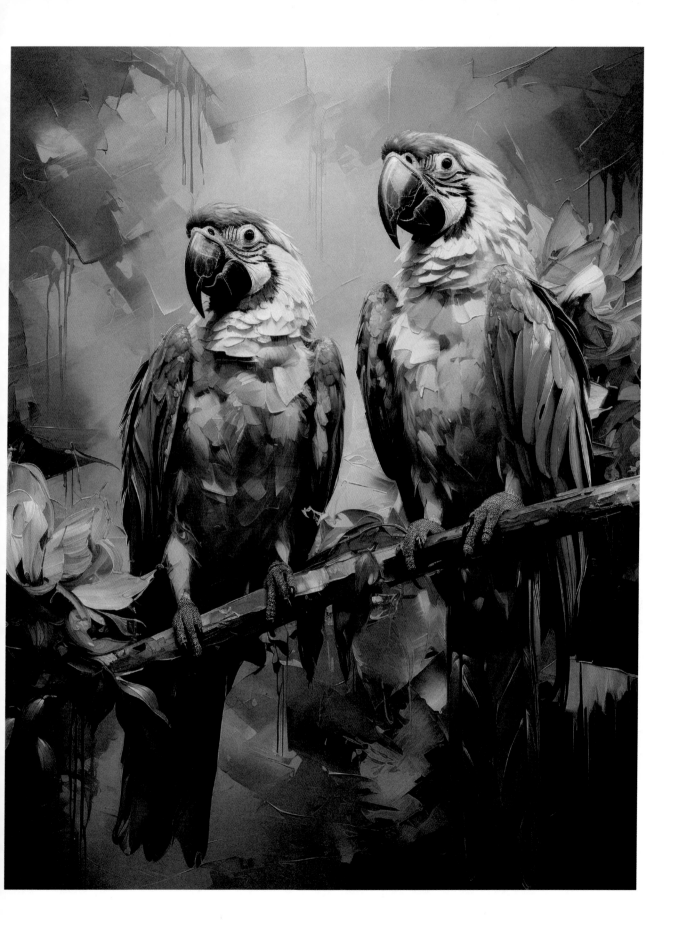

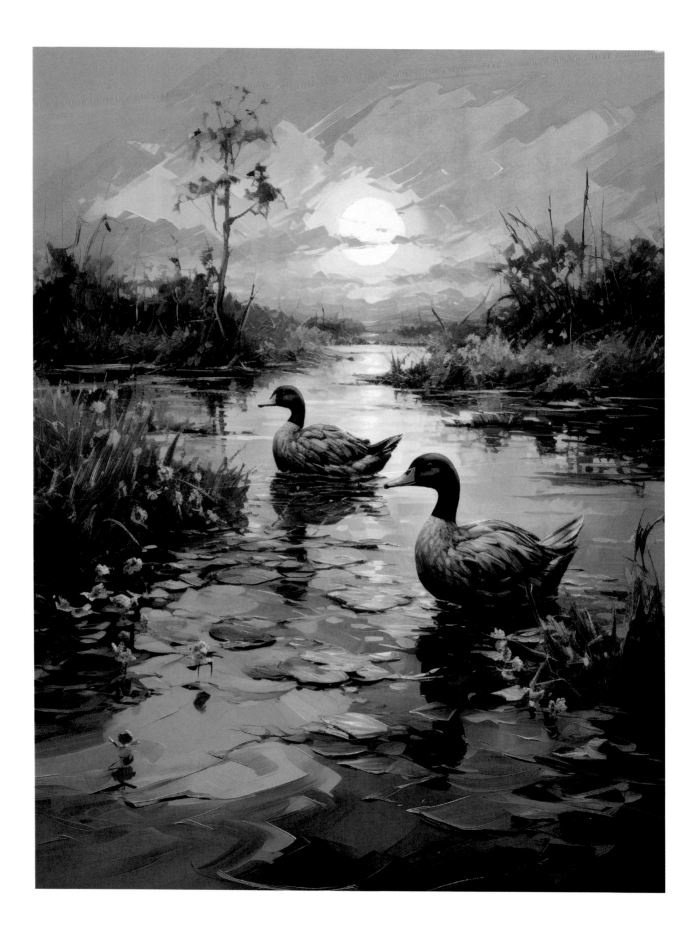

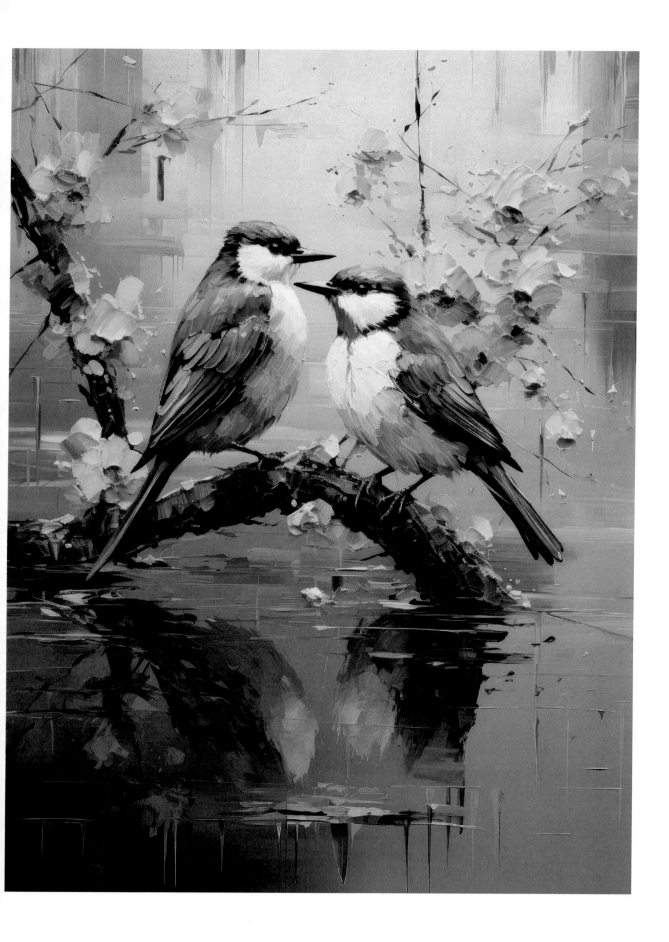

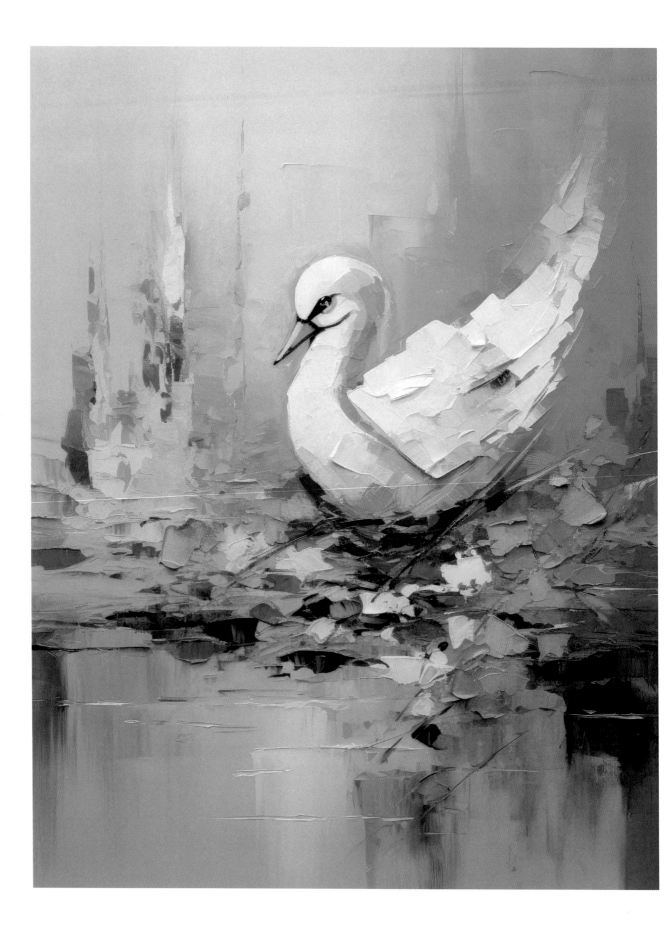

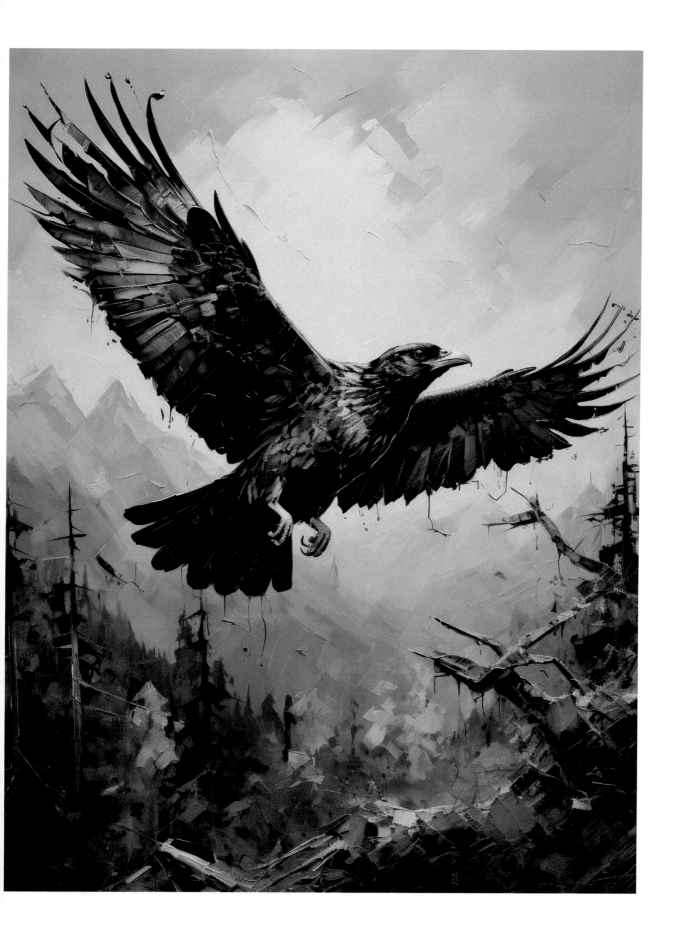

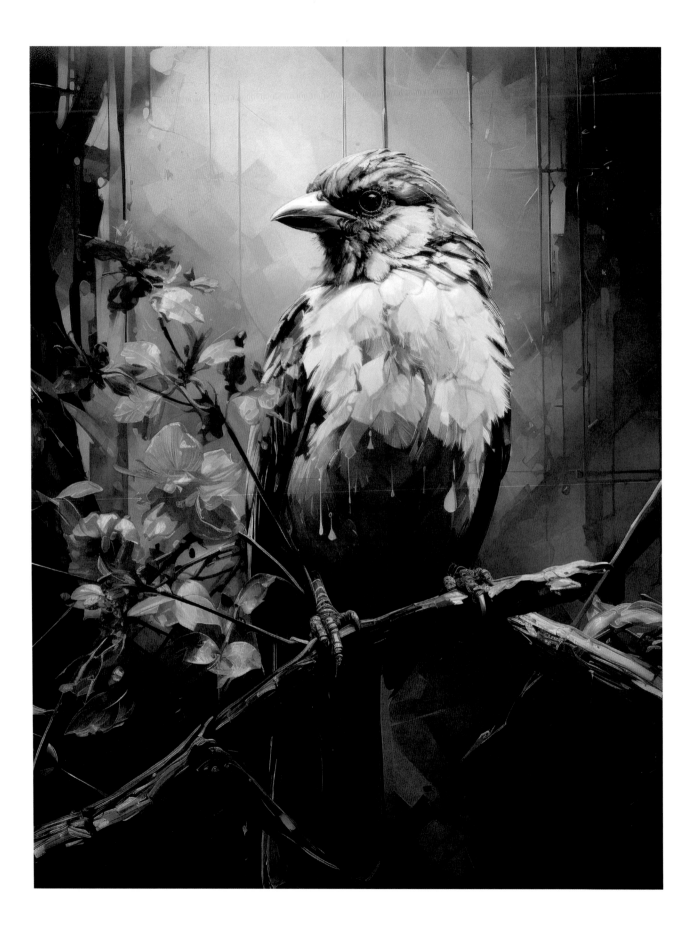

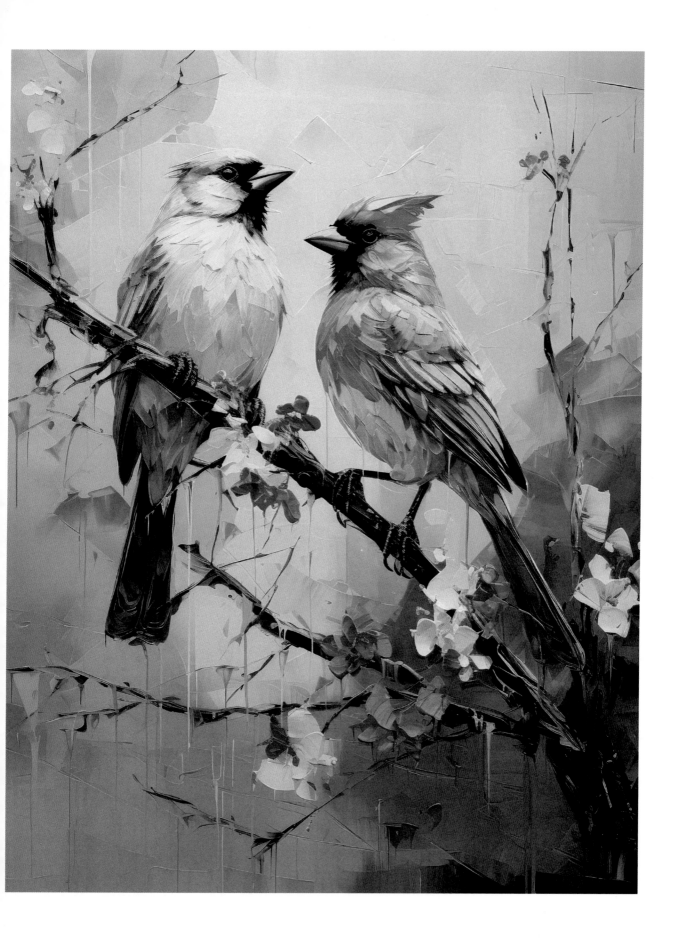

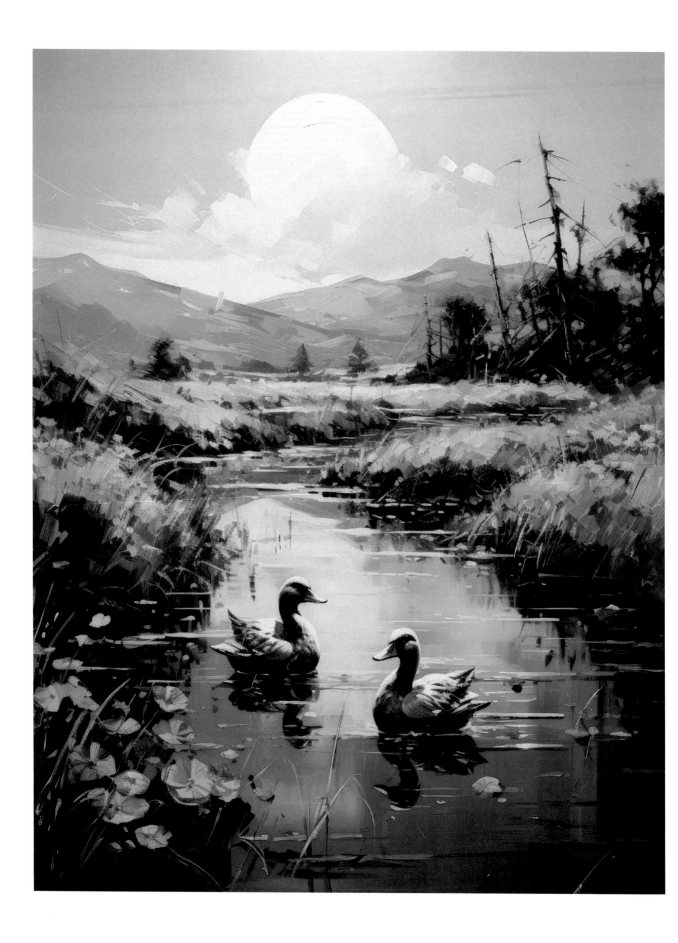

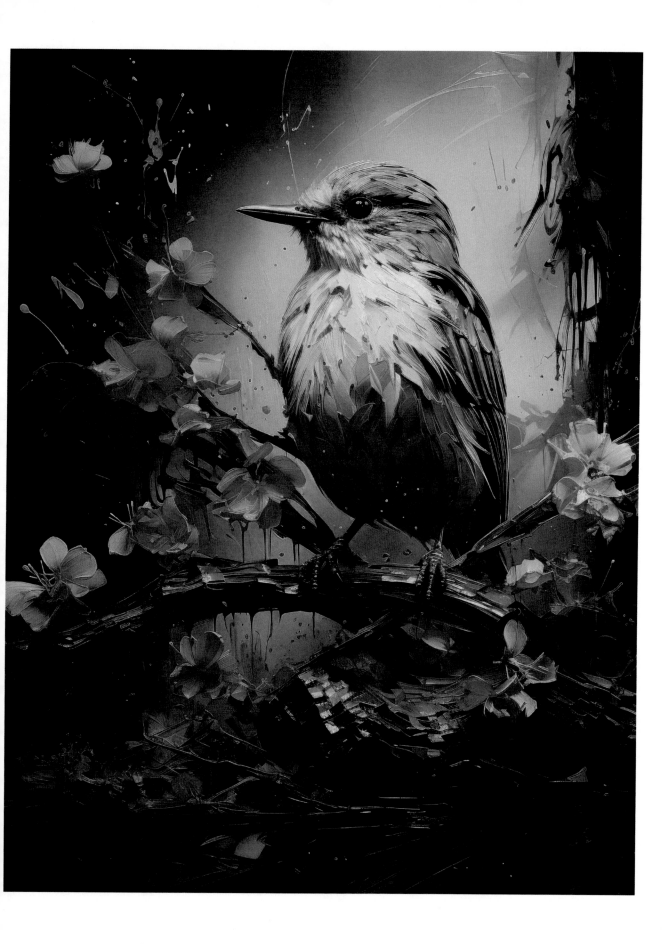

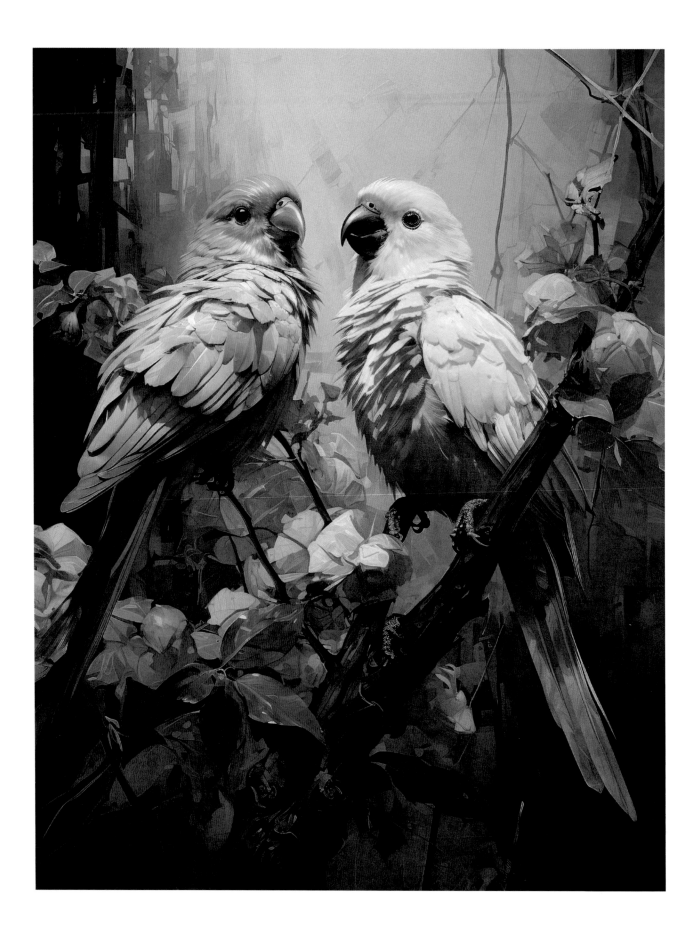

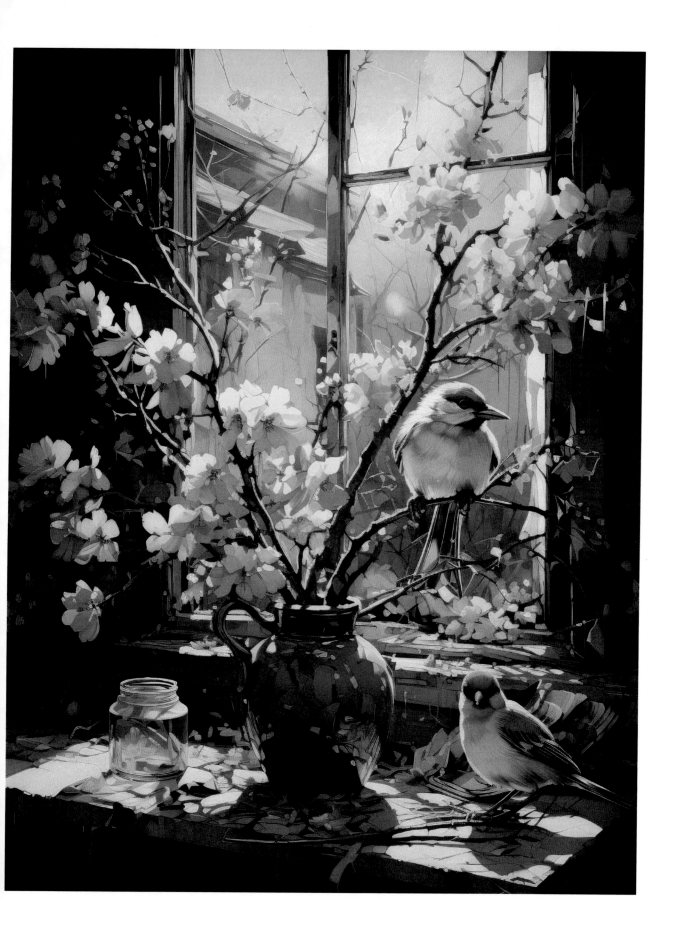

Thank you

Thanks for your interest in our books.

Please consider purchasing our other books
available now at Amazon.com.

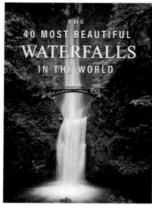
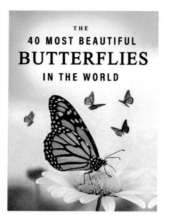
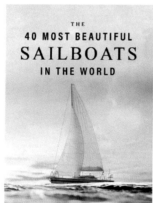
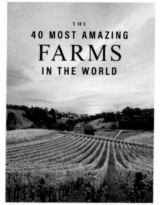

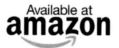

(Just search for "Blue Clover Books" on Amazon.)

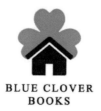

BLUE CLOVER
BOOKS

Made in the USA
Coppell, TX
18 November 2024

40445789R10062